Edward Gottheil, MD, PhD
Barry Stimmel, MD
Editors

Intensive Outpatient Treatment for the Addictions

Pre-publication
REVIEWS,
COMMENTARIES,
EVALUATIONS . . .

"This book provides a rich source of descriptive and effectiveness data for the newest drug abuse treatment modality, Intensive Outpatient Programs (IOP). While clinical books on such programs have previously appeared, this is the first book that focuses on IOP outcomes, including outcome comparisons with more traditional outpatient programs. The book contains several methodologically sophisticated, up-to-date research studies on IOP effectiveness. This book is a useful critical review of the state of the art in IOP, and provides a solid base for continuing research on IOP. Clinicians and researchers will find this book to be an invaluable source of up-to-date information on important issues relating to IOP, including the active ingredients of successful IOP, the effectiveness of IOP, causes of early drop-out, and the impact of psychiatric status and motivation for change on outcomes for patients. This book provides a foundation for the continuing development of the important Intensive Outpatient Treatment modality. The editor is a pioneer and key researcher in the IOP modality, the contributors are leading clinician-researchers. This innovative book will set the standard for all future research in the IOP modality. The book is essential reading for all clinicians and researchers committed to the improvement of Intensive Outpatient Treatment."

Stephen Magura, PhD
Director, Institute for Treatment Research, National Development and Research Institutes, Inc., New York

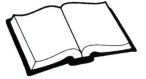

Intensive Outpatient Treatment for the Addictions

The *Journal of Addictive Diseases* series:*
(formerly *Advances in Alcohol & Substance Abuse* series)
- *Behavioral and Biochemical Issues in Substance Abuse**
- *Cocaine, AIDS, and Intravenous Drug Use**
- *What Works in Drug Abuse Epidemiology**
- *Cocaine: Physiological and Physiopathological Effects**
- *Comorbidity of Addictive and Psychiatric Disorders**
- *Experimental Therapeutics in Addiction Medicine**
- *The Effectiveness of Social Interventions for Homeless Substance Abusers**
- *The Neurobiology of Cocaine Addiction: From Bench to Bedside**
- *Intensive Outpatient Treatment for the Addictions**
- *Recent Advances in the Biology of Alcoholism*
- *The Effects of Maternal Alcohol and Drug Abuse on the Newborn*
- *Evaluation of Drug Treatment Programs*
- *Current Controversies in Alcoholism*
- *Federal Priorities in Funding Alcohol and Drug Abuse Programs*
- *Psychosocial Constructs of Alcoholism and Substance Abuse*
- *The Addictive Behaviors*
- *Conceptual Issues in Alcoholism and Substance Abuse*
- *Dual Addiction: Pharmacological Issues in the Treatment of Concomitant Alcoholism and Drug Abuse*
- *Cultural and Sociological Aspects of Alcoholism and Substance Abuse*
- *Alcohol and Drug Abuse in the Affluent*
- *Alcohol and Substance Abuse in Adolescence*
- *Controversies in Alcoholism and Substance Abuse*
- *Alcohol and Substance Abuse in Women and Children*
- *Cocaine: Pharmacology, Addiction, and Therapy*
- *Children of Alcoholics*
- *Pharmacological Issues in Alcohol and Substance Abuse*
- *AIDS and Substance Abuse*
- *Alcohol Research from Bench to Bedside*
- *Addiction Potential of Abused Drugs and Drug Classes*

Intensive Outpatient Treatment for the Addictions

Edward Gottheil, MD, PhD
Editor

Barry Stimmel, MD
Series Editor

HMP

The Haworth Medical Press
An Imprint of
The Haworth Press, Inc.
New York • London

Published by

The Haworth Medical Press, 10 Alice Street, Binghamton, NY 13904-1580 USA

The Haworth Medical Press is an imprint of The Haworth Press, Inc., 10 Alice Street, Binghamton, NY 13904-1580 USA.

Intensive Outpatient Treatment for the Addictions has also been published as *Journal of Addictive Diseases*, Volume 16, Number 2 1997.

Cover design: Thomas J. Mayshock Jr.

Library of Congress Cataloging-in-Publication Data

Intensive outpatient treatment for the addictions / Edward Gottheil, editor; Barry Stimmel, series editor.

       p. cm.–(Journal of addictive diseases; v. 16, no. 2)
       Includes bibliographical references and index.
       ISBN 0-7890-0313-9 (alk. paper)
       1. Alcoholism–Treatment. 2. Drug abuse–Treatment. 3. Ambulatory medical care. I. Gottheil, Edward L. II. Stimmel, Barry, 1939-   . IIII. Series.
       [DNLM: 1. Substance Dependence–therapy. 2. Ambulatory Care. 3. Substance Abuse Treatment Centers–organization & administration. W1 JO533PU v. 16 no. 2 1997 / WM 270 I6015 1997]
RC564.7.I58 1997
616.86'06–dc21
DNLM/DLC   97-3576
for Library of Congress   CIP

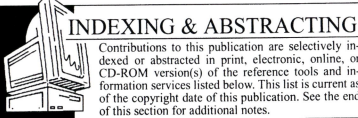

INDEXING & ABSTRACTING

Contributions to this publication are selectively indexed or abstracted in print, electronic, online, or CD-ROM version(s) of the reference tools and information services listed below. This list is current as of the copyright date of this publication. See the end of this section for additional notes.

- *Abstracts in Anthropology,* Baywood Publishing Company, 26 Austin Avenue, P.O. Box 337, Amityville, NY 11701

- *Abstracts of Research in Pastoral Care & Counseling,* Loyola College, 7135 Minstrel Way, Suite 101, Columbia, MD 21045

- *Academic Abstracts/CD-ROM,* EBSCO Publishing Editorial Department, P.O. Box 590, Ipswich, MA 01938-0590

- *ADDICTION ABSTRACTS,* National Addiction Centre, 4 Windsor Walk, London SE5 8AF, England

- *ALCONLINE Database,* Swedish Council for Information on Alcohol and Other Drugs, Box 27302, S-102 54 Stockholm, Sweden

- *Behavioral Medicine Abstracts,* University of Washington, School of Social Work, Seattle, WA 98195

- *Biosciences Information Service of Biological Abstracts (BIOSIS),* Biosciences Information Service, 2100 Arch Street, Philadelphia, PA 19103-1399

- *Brown University Digest of Addiction Theory and Application, The (DATA Newsletter),* Project Cork Institute, Dartmouth Medical School, 14 South Main Street, Suite 2F, Hanover, NH 03755-2015

- *Cambridge Scientific Abstracts,* Health & Safety Science Abstracts, Environmental Routenet (accessed via INTERNET), 7200 Wisconsin Avenue #601, Bethesda, MD 20814

- *Child Development Abstracts & Bibliography,* University of Kansas, 2 Bailey Hall, Lawrence, KS 66045

- *CNPIEC Reference Guide: Chinese National Directory of Foreign Periodicals,* P.O. Box 88, Beijing, Peoples Republic of China

- *Criminal Justice Abstracts,* Willow Tree Press, 15 Washington Street, 4th Floor, Newark, NJ 07102

- *Criminal Justice Periodical Index,* University Microfilms, Inc., 300 North Zeeb Road, Ann Arbor, MI 48106

(continued)

- *Criminology, Penology and Police Science Abstracts,* Kugler Publications, P.O. Box 11188, 1001 GD Amsterdam, The Netherlands
- *Current Contents . . . .* see: *Institute for Scientific Information*
- *Educational Administration Abstracts (EAA),* Sage Publications, Inc., 2455 Teller Road, Newbury Park, CA 91320
- *Excerpta Medica/Secondary Publishing Division,* Elsevier Science Inc., Secondary Publishing Division, 655 Avenue of the Americas, New York, NY 10010
- *Family Studies Database (online and CD/ROM),* National Information Services Corporation, 306 East Baltimore Pike, 2nd Floor, Media, PA 19063
- *Health Source: Indexing & Abstracting of 160 selected health related journals, updated monthly,* EBSCO Publishing, 83 Pine Street, Peabody, MA 01960
- *Health Source Plus: expanded version of "Health Source" to be released shortly:* EBSCO Publishing, 83 Pine Street, Peabody, MA 01960
- *Index Medicus,* National Library of Medicine, 8600 Rockville Pike, Bethesda, MD 20894
- *Index to Periodical Articles Related to Law,* University of Texas, 727 East 26th Street, Austin, TX 78705
- *Institute for Scientific Information,* 3501 Market Street, Philadelphia, Pennsylvania 19104. Coverage in:
  a) Social Science Citation Index (SSCI): print, online, CD-ROM
  b) Research Alerts (current awareness service)
  c) Social SciSearch (magnetic tape)
  d) Current Contents/Social & Behavioral Sciences (weekly current awareness service)
- *International Pharmaceutical Abstracts,* ASHP, 7272 Wisconsin Avenue, Bethesda, MD 20814
- *INTERNET ACCESS (& additional networks) Bulletin Board for Libraries ("BUBL"), coverage of information resources on INTERNET, JANET, and other networks.*
  - JANET X.29: UK.AC.BATH.BUBL or 00006012101300
  - TELNET: BUBL.BATH.AC.UK or 138.38.32.45 login 'bubl'
  - Gopher: BUBL.BATH.AC.UK (138.32.32.45). Port 7070
  - World Wide Web: http: / / www.bubl.bath.ac.uk./BUBL/ home.html
  - NISSWAIS: telnetniss.ac.uk (for the NISS gateway)
  The Andersonian Library, Curran Building, 101 St. James Road, Glasgow G4 ONS, Scotland
- *Medication Use STudies (MUST) Database,* The University of Mississippi, School of Pharmacy, University, MS 38677

(continued)

- *Mental Health Abstracts (online through DIALOG),* IFI/Plenum Data Company, 3202 Kirkwood Highway, Wilmington, DE 19808

- *NIAAA Alcohol and Alcohol Problems Science Database (ETOH),* National Institute on Alcohol Abuse and Alcoholism, 1400 Eye Street NW, Suite 600, Washington, DC 20005

- *PASCAL International Bibliography T205: Sciences de l'information Documentation,* INIST/CNRS-Service Gestion des Documents Primaires, 2 allee du Parc de Brabois, F-54514 Vandoeuvre-les-Nancy, Cedex, France

- *Psychological Abstracts (PsycINFO),* American Psychological Association, P.O. Box 91600, Washington, DC 20090-1600

- *Sage Family Studies Abstracts (SFSA),* Sage Publications, Inc., 2455 Teller Road, Newbury Park, CA 91320

- *Sage Urban Studies Abstracts (SUSA),* Sage Publications, Inc., 2455 Teller Road, Newbury Park, CA 91320

- *Social Planning/Policy & Development Abstracts (SOPODA),* Sociological Abstracts, Inc., P.O. Box 22206, San Diego, CA 92192-0206

- *Social Work Abstracts,* National Association of Social Workers, 750 First Street NW, 8th Floor, Washington, DC 20002

- *Sociological Abstracts (SA),* Sociological Abstracts, Inc., P.O. Box 22206, San Diego, CA 92192-0206

- *SOMED (social medicine) Database,* Landes Institut fur Den Offentlichen Gesundheitsdienst NRW, Postfach 20 10 12, D-33548 Bielefeld, Germany

- *Studies on Women Abstracts,* Carfax Publishing Company, P.O. Box 25, Abingdon, Oxfordshire, OX14 3UE, United Kingdom

- *Violence and Abuse Abstracts: A Review of Current Literature on Interpersonal Violence (VAA),* Sage Publications, Inc., 2455 Teller Road, Newbury Park, CA 91320

(continued)

SPECIAL BIBLIOGRAPHIC NOTES

related to special journal issues (separates)
and indexing/abstracting

❏ indexing/abstracting services in this list will also cover material in any "separate" that is co-published simultaneously with Haworth's special thematic journal issue or DocuSerial. Indexing/abstracting usually covers material at the article/chapter level.

❏ monographic co-editions are intended for either non-subscribers or libraries which intend to purchase a second copy for their circulating collections.

❏ monographic co-editions are reported to all jobbers/wholesalers/approval plans. The source journal is listed as the "series" to assist the prevention of duplicate purchasing in the same manner utilized for books-in-series.

❏ to facilitate user/access services all indexing/abstracting services are encouraged to utilize the co-indexing entry note indicated at the bottom of the first page of each article/chapter/contribution.

❏ this is intended to assist a library user of any reference tool (whether print, electronic, online, or CD-ROM) to locate the monographic version if the library has purchased this version but not a subscription to the source journal.

❏ individual articles/chapters in any Haworth publication are also available through the Haworth Document Delivery Services (HDDS).

Intensive Outpatient Treatment for the Addictions

CONTENTS

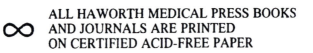

ALL HAWORTH MEDICAL PRESS BOOKS
AND JOURNALS ARE PRINTED
ON CERTIFIED ACID-FREE PAPER

ABOUT THE EDITOR

Edward Gottheil, MD, PhD, is Professor of Psychiatry and Human Behavior at Jefferson Medical College of Thomas Jefferson University in Philadelphia, Pennsylvania, where he is also Director of Alcohol and Drug Abuse Services and an attending psychiatrist. Dr. Gottheil is Associate Editor of *Recent Developments in Alcoholism* and a member of the editorial boards for *The American Journal of Drug and Alcohol Abuse* and *Substance Abuse*. He is Chair of the Biopsychological Research Committee of the American Academy of Psychiatrists in Alcoholism & Addictions and a member of the Board of Directors of the American Academy of Addiction Psychiatry. Dr. Gottheil has also served as principal investigator for several funded programs: currently he is involved in ongoing research with the Delaware State Hospital Research Unit. He has co-edited six books and over 140 journal articles on substance abuse, addiction, and treatment.

EDITORIALS

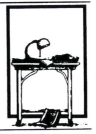

Intensive Outpatient Treatment: Methods and Outcomes

Four of the six papers in this issue were presented at the 1995 ASAM Symposium on Intensive Outpatient Treatment. They include: a general history and introduction,[1] a program description and

Address correspondence to: Edward Gottheil, MD, PhD, Department of Psychiatry, Jefferson Medical College, 1201 Chestnut Street, 15th Floor, Philadelphia, PA 19107.

This research was supported in part by Grant #1 R18 DA 06166 from the National Institute on Drug Abuse and performed under the auspices of the Commonwealth Office of Drug and Alcohol Programs and the Philadelphia Department of Public Health, Coordinating Office for Drug and Alcohol Abuse Programs. Its contents are solely the responsibility of the authors and do not necessarily represent the official views of the awarding agencies NIDA, ODAP, and CODAAP.

[Haworth co-indexing entry note]: "Intensive Outpatient Treatment: Methods and Outcomes." Gottheil, Edward. Co-published simultaneously in *Journal of Addictive Diseases* (The Haworth Medical Press, an imprint of The Haworth Press, Inc.) Vol. 16, No. 2, 1997, pp. xv-xix; and: *Intensive Outpatient Treatment for the Addictions* (ed: Edward Gottheil, and Barry Stimmel) The Haworth Medical Press, an imprint of The Haworth Press, Inc., 1997, pp. xiii-xvii Single or multiple copies of this article are available for a fee from The Haworth Document Delivery Service [1-800-342-9678, 9:00 a.m. - 5:00 p.m. (EST). E-mail address: getinfo@haworth.com].

follow-up,[2] a comparison with individual outpatient counseling,[3] and a comparison of 6 intensive with 10 traditional outpatient programs.[4] The other two papers include one on early dropouts[5] and one on follow-up.[6] Together, these papers provide descriptions, discussions, and to the best of my knowledge, the first outcome evaluations of the new intensive outpatient treatment modality.

In 1982, Washton[1] started a cocaine addiction IOP (intensive outpatient program), perhaps the first of its kind in the nation, and "not a single third party payer would reimburse us for the program." IOP was not a recognized term back then, much less an approved modality. In 1988, when the number of cocaine abusers requesting treatment grew beyond what the capacity of the existing substance abuse treatment system in Philadelphia could accommodate (as was true elsewhere in the country), funds were requested and obtained to support a new Jefferson outpatient cocaine treatment program. The question then was how to treat these patients. A review of the literature at that time indicated that many psychosocial and pharmacological therapies had been tried but that no preferred treatment for cocaine dependence had emerged. However, a number of programs were beginning to try more intensive outpatient treatment approaches which appeared clinically promising. Despite the fact that the medical assistance system of Pennsylvania did not then and does not now recognize IOPs or reimburse them, it seemed worth trying a version of the approach, which is described by Weinstein et al.[3] later in this volume. Apparently, many others came to the same conclusion and the number of intensive outpatient programs increased greatly. In less than a decade IOP has become an important treatment modality and a widely accepted level of care. It is considered a treatment of choice for many substance dependent patients and its popularity continues to grow as clinicians seem to believe in its helpfulness. Nevertheless, there have been no reported controlled studies of its effectiveness which is what prompted us to organize the ASAM symposium.

Washton, in his presentation, provided an interesting history of and perspective on the development of the IOP. Drawing on his long experience, he also described for us 10 important ingredients which he believes are intrinsic to the delivery of effective IOP treatment.

One of the rationales for implementing more intensive outpatient treatment programs was the hope that it might help reduce early treatment dropouts, a persistent problem for substance abuse programs.[5] Since many patients enter treatment on impulse rather than resolve, traditional weekly visits may allow too much time for temptation, vacillation and relapse to occur. More frequent visits could lead to earlier engagement and commitment to continue in the program. Early dropouts, however, are not well studied as they are often excluded from treatment comparisons in which the goal is to compare patients who have received some specified number of the intended treatments rather than those leaving with little or no treatment exposure. These early dropouts were the focus of the paper by Gottheil et al.[5] who compared the intake characterisitcs and 9-month follow-up outcomes of cocaine dependent outpatient admissions who dropped out during intake and prior to receiving one treatment service, with those who returned for at least one therapy visit, and those who remained in treatment for two months or more.

The structure and functioning of a model of intensive outpatient program for cocaine dependent patients was described in close to "how-to" detail by Campbell et al.[2] Of 151 patients in that program included in a 6-month follow-up study, only 36 had no diagnoses in addition to cocaine dependence; 57 had two or more. The main results of the study were that (a) no relationship was found between diagnostic groupings and retention, and (b) significant improvement was demonstrated by reductions in scores on the composite scales of the ASI. In similar vein, Campbell[6] found that 77% of patients admitted to a half-way house in Canada reported being drug free in three months. These patients also demonstrated improvement by reductions in ASI composite scale scores. Interestingly, assessment of readiness for change stage at intake was not found to be related to outcome. Campbell et al.[2] concluded that while IOP for crack cocaine-dependent patients was efficacious, controlled comparisons with inpatient and with standard outpatient programs were needed.

The findings of a five year randomized, controlled study comparing intensive outpatient treatment with more standard individual counseling and with individual plus once-weekly group treatment were reported by Weinstein et al.[3] It is perhaps worth noting that the study took place in a publicly supported, community based, urban clinic. In-treatment and end-of-treatment assessments revealed marked improvement for each of the treatment groups, with those persons remaining in treatment longest showing the most improvement. However, the results of this random assignment, clinical trial revealed no significant differences on any of the assessments between the new intensive outpatient treatment modality and the more traditional modalities.

In the last paper, McLellan et al.[4] compared the intake characteristics, treatment services received, and outcomes of patients in 6 samples of intensive outpatient programs and 10 samples of traditional outpatient programs. The program samples were selected according to explicit definitional criteria from their national database of "real world" treatment programs. At six-month follow-up, patients in both modalities were found to have improved significantly, but there were few differences between the IOP and traditional modalities.

There has been considerable concern about the research-clinical gap, the need for knowledge transfer from "bench to trench," and the time and problem of translating the knowledge into clinical practice. There are also clinical-research gaps. Based on clinical observations and papers, IOP seemed to be helpful and grew rapidly to become common practice. This growth, however, occurred without significant research support. Indeed, the first comparisons of IOP and more traditional programs in the papers by Weinstein et al. and McLellan et al. did not show IOP to be superior to traditional outpatient programs. These are but two studies, however, and there are many possible variations of IOP. Intensive programs may differ with respect to frequency of visits, length of visits, duration of the treatment programs, supportive vs. dynamic approach, behavioral vs. nondirective approach, and number and varieties of therapies offered. There really would seem to be a need to conduct many more controlled comparisons of different IOP programs with traditional programs. The important question in all likelihood will not be whether IOP or traditional is better, but will again revert to the matching problem of which patients do better in which variations of IOP and traditional programs. At present, IOP is well established clinically, but the research story remains to be told.

Edward Gottheil, MD, PhD
Department of Psychiatry and Human Behavior
Thomas Jefferson University
Philadelphia, PA 19107

REFERENCES

1. Washton AM. Evolution of intensive outpatient treatment (IOP) as a "legitimate" treatment modality. Editorial. J Addict Dis. 1997; 16(2): xix-xxv.

2. Campbell J, Gabrielli W, Laster LJ, Liskow BI. Efficacy of outpatient intensive treatment for drug abuse. J Addict Dis. 1997; 16(2): 15-25.

3. Weinstein SP, Gottheil E, Sterling RC. Randomized comparison of intensive outpatient vs. individual therapy for cocaine abusers. J Addict Dis. 1997; 16(2): 41-56.

4. McLellan AT, Hagan TA, Meyers K, Randall M, Durell J. "Intensive" outpatient substance abuse treatment: comparisons with "traditional" outpatient treatment. J Addict Dis. 1997; 16(2): 57-85.

5. Gottheil E, Sterling RC, Weinstein SP. Pretreatment dropouts: characteristics and outcomes. J Addict Dis. 1997; 16(2): 1-14.

6. Campbell WG. Evaluation of a residential program using the addiction severity index and stages of change. J Addict Dis. 1997; 16(2): 27-39.

Evolution
of Intensive Outpatient Treatment (IOP)
as a "Legitimate" Treatment Modality

My experience with outpatient treatment of alcohol and substance abuse spans across the past 21 years and has included work in both public and private facilities, hospital-based and free-standing facilities, programs that were designed exclusively for either heroin addicts, alcoholics, or cocaine/crack addicts, as well as integrated programs capable of treating all types of chemical dependencies regardless of the patient's drug of choice. During these years I have seen intensive outpatient treatment (IOP) evolve from a scarcely available and poorly respected modality into the preferred treatment for many who seek professional help for chemical dependency. I have seen it develop from aftercare to primary care; from a nonreimbursed and poorly understood service to a treatment of first choice by managed care and other third-party payers.[1,2]

In the 1970's, while working in a heroin addiction outpatient treatment clinic in East Harlem, I learned firsthand the importance of providing easy access to primary outpatient care for opioid addicts who either could not gain admission to inpatient care and/or preferred not to leave their home, family, and/or job as a requirement of receiving treatment. The inpatient detoxification unit originally connected to this outpatient program lost its funding and closed down in the early '70s. This gave our clinical and research staffs additional impetus to do everything possible to maximize the

[Haworth co-indexing entry note]: "Evolution of Intensive Outpatient Treatment (IOP) as a 'Legitimate' Treatment Modality." Washton, Arnold M. Co-published simultaneously in *Journal of Addictive Diseases* (The Haworth Medical Press, an imprint of The Haworth Press, Inc.) Vol. 16, No. 2, 1997, pp. xxi-xxvii; and: *Intensive Outpatient Treatment for the Addictions* (ed: Edward Gottheil, and Barry Stimmel) The Haworth Medical Press, an imprint of The Haworth Press, Inc., 1997, pp. xix-xxv. Single or multiple copies of this article are available for a fee from The Haworth Document Delivery Service [1-800-342-9678, 9:00 a.m. - 5:00 p.m. (EST). E-mail address: getinfo@haworth.com].

efficacy of outpatient care, including combining psychosocial interventions with various investigational pharmacotherapies. We were among the first, for example, to utilize clonidine to facilitate opioid withdrawal, naltrexone to facilitate relapse prevention, and LAAM (l-alpha acetyl methadol) to facilitate opioid maintenance in an outpatient setting.[3,4,5] Despite a fair amount of success in these efforts, our outpatient programs were often viewed as less desirable and less effective than long-term residential care. At that time the prevailing attitude among many workers in the field and among the public at large was that addicts must be removed from their drug-using environment (and preferably for a very long time) in order to be meaningfully rehabilitated. Outpatient treatment was seen as a poor alternative to extended residential care.

Of all the forces that have accelerated the evolution of IOP as a "legitimate" treatment modality, the cocaine epidemic of the 1980's is perhaps the most significant.[1,2] Cocaine snorters were literally flooding a treatment system which was prepared to deal only with heroin addicts or alcoholics. Cocaine-specific treatment was simply unavailable at that time since most treatment centers were taken off guard by the rapid influx of this new "breed" of addict. Early in the cocaine epidemic, most who sought treatment were white, middle-class, employed, drug-sophisticated, entitled, and had no history of prior treatment for addiction. Unlike heroin addicts they neither demanded nor required pharmacologic withdrawal or medication. Unlike alcoholics they were using an illicit substance and typically showed no serious (health-threatening) medical problems related to their use. In most cases, there were no medical indications for hospitalization. Moreover, most preferred to be treated as outpatients since they did not want to leave their job and/or family. They were also concerned about the social stigma associated with being "sent away" to a drug rehab or psychiatric hospital for treatment. They preferred to be treated in a private rather than public facility, but they were clearly in need of more structured, addiction-specific treatment than solo practitioners (e.g, therapists) were equipped to offer. Hence, the emerging need for and subsequent proliferation of private programs offering intensive outpatient treatment.

In 1982, I started a specialized cocaine addiction IOP in Manhattan (perhaps one of the first of its kind in the nation) and although the patients found it to be very conducive to their needs not a single third party payer would reimburse us for the program. Insurance reimbursement at that time was available only for inpatient but not outpatient addiction care. Structured outpatient treatment was categorically excluded from reimbursement as a primary modality of addiction care. In certain cases IOP was eligible for reimbursement only if provided as aftercare immediately following an episode of inpatient treatment. When faced with the choice of paying out-of-pocket for outpatient treatment versus receiving full coverage for inpatient treatment, it was no surprise that many clients chose inpatient over outpatient treatment even when inpatient care was not necessary for clinical reasons alone. Apart from this topsy-turvy reimbursement structure, there was still a pervasive sense among many treatment professionals (especially those with a strong 12-step orientation) that in order to be truly effective, treatment must start with a 28-day or longer inpatient stay. The net result of all of this was that outpatient treatment continued to be seen by many as merely aftercare rather than legitimate primary care.

The most recent boost to acceptance of IOP as a truly legitimate treatment modality has come from the proliferation of managed care with its attendant focus on cost-containment and cost-effectiveness. Patient placement and utilization management criteria developed by managed care companies typically direct treatment toward the most clinically appropriate and least restrictive environment. In general, this means that in the absence of serious risk factors (e.g., active suicidality/homicidality, psychosis, withdrawal complications, chronic relapse) patients are referred for treatment to outpatient rather than inpatient facilities. To some extent, managed care has had a free hand to develop their own criteria because the research literature is inconsistent and inconclusive regarding the efficacy of inpatient versus outpatient approaches in addicted populations. The esteemed panel of researchers who follow me in this symposium will surely address this issue in greater detail.

All in all, in the era of managed care IOP has become the treatment of first choice for clients who present with alcohol and/or drug problems unless there are specific clinical indications for a higher (more intensive or restrictive) level of care. The availability of IOP has also allowed managed care to shorten inpatient stays knowing that the client can be "stepped down" to a highly structured outpatient program where the client will be closely followed upon discharge. Obviously, this situation represents a complete turnabout from the past when IOP was largely ignored or just not thought of as a legitimate modality that warranted reimbursement.

Despite the recent recognition of IOP as a legitimate modality, it is certainly not the most appropriate treatment modality for all addicted clients (nor is any other modality) and identification of patients most likely to benefit from IOP remains a challenge. At present, the decision to refer/admit a client to IOP is based more on exclusion of those who are clearly inappropriate for this level of care (based largely on risk factors as mentioned above) than on identification of specific factors that predict who will do well in such a program. Psychiatric risk factors aside, it appears that the patients who do best in IOP are those who can get themselves to show up reliably for scheduled sessions and put into action the basic nuts-and-bolts behavioral changes (e.g., avoid relapse triggers, utilize support systems, develop alternative activities, practice thought stopping and craving control techniques, etc.) that are required to establish and maintain abstinence in the "real world" where access to drugs/alcohol is ever-present and so are the cues and pressures (both internal and external) to use these substances. It is often impossible to predict which patients are "motivated" enough to make good use of an IOP until they have actually been given a chance to participate in the program. I have seen many examples of patients who do well in IOP despite a history of chronic relapse and previous treatment failures. Eligibility for IOP should not be ruled out solely based on the client' treatment history alone. As IOP has proliferated, programs have expanded their ability to treat a wider range of patients, especially programs that have incorporated psychiatric services into their service-delivery configuration. It is not uncommon these days to find specialized dual-diagnosis components within an IOP for patients who have co-existing psychiatric and chemical dependency disorders.

In the absence of consistent research findings that can tell us definitively what factors contribute to the success or effectiveness of IOP in a given patient population, I will take the liberty afforded me to speak from my own clinical experience and outline what I feel are ten of the most important factors that contribute to the success of intensive outpatient treatment:[6]

1. *Treat your patients as valued customers.* Make sure that your entire staff, from receptionists to counselors and physicians, deal courteously and respectfully with patients, no matter what!

2. *Be flexible in the delivery of your services.* There is no boiler plate program that has been shown to be more effective than others. Adjusting the program to the patients rather than vice versa, is absolutely essential.

3. *Do supervised urine testing on all patients at least twice per week.* Urine testing is an invaluable clinical tool that can help patients control their cravings and impulses to use. It is also an objective measure of treatment progress. Never use urine testing as a police tactic to try to catch patients in a lie. Use it as a clinical tool to enhance treatment effectiveness.

4. *Schedule frequent sessions at the beginning of treatment.* Frequency rather than duration of visits is more important on the front end. Seeing a patient 4-5 times per week at first can be helpful in getting a good therapeutic alliance started and creating an "environment of safety."

5. *Provide psychoeducation about addiction, recovery, and relapse, but be careful not to make this the centerpiece of the program and make sure that it is carefully integrated with other services.* There is no evidence that the chances of successful recovery are enhanced by providing patients with a college-level course in "Addiction 101." Too much didactic information may overshadow and displace more important issues and day-to-day struggles that patients must be given an opportunity to address.

6. *Deal with slips as motivational crises rather than mistakes.* Slips should be viewed as behavioral manifestations of the patient's ambivalence about giving up alcohol/drugs. A slip is evidence of the internal struggle between the forces that want to stop using and those that do not. Reframing slips in this way can help to better identify what is causing the continued use and how best to stop it.

7. *Encourage but do not mandate patient involvement in 12-step*

and/or other self-help programs. Trying to coerce clients into accepting AA, NA, CA, or other forms of self-help is likely to backfire. These and other heavy-handed tactics often promote rather than prevent early dropout from treatment. It is often better to encourage self-help involvement by educating patients about the positive attributes of self-help and by utilizing a buddy-system in which patients who are further along in their treatment and already meaningfully involved in self-help volunteer to escort one or more newcomers to meetings. Patients who initially refuse to attend self-help should not be made to feel that they are "failing" in treatment, especially if they are remaining abstinent.

8. *Divide the program into sequential phases.* This affords a more concentrated approach for patients in each phase of recovery and also provides a concrete marker of progress as patients "graduate" or progress from one phase of treatment to the next. It can also enhance patient-treatment matching. For example, patients who are mandated or coerced into treatment may require motivational counseling to work through their resentments and ambivalence before being ready to make use of an early abstinence program that presumes that patients admit that they have a chemical dependency problem and agree to try total abstinence as a first step. Similarly, patients who have established stable abstinence and improved their psychosocial functioning should have an opportunity to receive relapse prevention counseling to help them maintain their progress.

9. *Insure continuity of care.* Wherever possible, the patient should be involved with the same primary counselor or case manager throughout the program. The less switching between counselors and groups the better. Continuity in caregivers tends to minimize opportunities for splitting and reduces precipitous dropout.

10. *Select your clinical staff very carefully.* A counselor's recovery status is irrelevant to how effective they are in treating addicts. Skilled clinicians who can be warm, empathetic, tolerant, nonjudgmental, flexible, focused, firm, and clear will be the most effective. Choose counselors who are good motivation mobilizers and change facilitators. These are people who like doing counseling and know how to talk to the patients with empathy and concern. They focus on patients' strengths rather than weaknesses. They are

eternal optimists and not easily frustrated. They maintain clear boundaries, but do not come across as distant. Staff selection may be the most critical variable of all in determining treatment effectiveness.

Arnold M. Washton, PhD, CSAC
The Washton Institute
New York, NY 10017

REFERENCES

1. Washton AM. Cocaine addiction: treatment recovery and relapse prevention. New York: Norton, 1989.

2. Washton AM. (Ed.). Psychotherapy and substance abuse: a practitioner's handbook. New York, Guilford, 1995.

3. Washton AM, Resnick RB. Clonidine for opiate detoxification: outpatient clinical trials. *American Journal of Psychiatry,* 137 (9): 1121-1122, 1980.

4. Resnick RB, Washton AM, Thomas MA, Kestenbaum RS. Naltrexone in the treatment of opiate dependence. In: RC Peterson (Ed.), International Challenge of Drug Abuse, NIDA Research Monograph No. 19, Department of Health, Education, and Welfare, Washington, DC, pp. 321-332, 1978.

5. Resnick RB, Washton AM, Garwood J, Perzel J. LAAM instead of take-home methadone. In: LS Harris (Ed.), Problems of drug dependence. NIDA Research Monograph No. 41, Department of Health and Human Services; Alcohol Drug Abuse, and Mental Health Administration, Rockville, Maryland, pp. 505-507, 1982.

6. Washton AM, Stone-Washton N. Intensive treatment of cocaine addiction: techniques to improve its effectiveness. *International Journal of the Addictions,* 25: 1421-1429, 1991.

Pretreatment Dropouts: Characteristics and Outcomes

Edward Gottheil, MD, PhD
Robert C. Sterling, PhD
Stephen P. Weinstein, PhD

SUMMARY. The characteristics and outcome results of 123 cocaine dependent patients who dropped out following intake without returning for even one treatment visit were compared with those of 324 who did return and received at least one treatment service and 118 who remained on the program for two months or more.

The pre-treatment dropouts were more often positive for cocaine on admission drug screens and less often employed. They reported fewer psychological symptoms on the scales of the SCL-90 and received lower scores on the medical problem severity scale of the ASI. At 9-month follow-up they were found to have less often at-

---

Edward Gottheil, Robert C. Sterling, and Stephen P. Weinstein are affiliated with Thomas Jefferson University, Department of Psychiatry and Human Behavior, Philadelphia, PA.

Address correspondence to: Edward Gottheil, MD, PhD, Department of Psychiatry, Jefferson Medical College, 1201 Chestnut Street, 15th Floor, Philadelphia, PA 19107.

This research was supported in part by Grant # 1 R18 DA 06166 from the National Institute on Drug Abuse and performed under the auspices of the Commonwealth Office of Drug and Alcohol Programs and the Philadelphia Department of Public Health, Coordinating Office for Drug and Alcohol Abuse Programs. Its contents are solely the responsibility of the authors and do not necessarily represent the official views of the awarding agencies NIDA, ODAP, and CODAAP.

[Haworth co-indexing entry note]: "Pretreatment Dropouts: Characteristics and Outcomes." Gottheil, Edward, Robert C. Sterling, and Stephen P. Weinstein. Co-published simultaneously in *Journal of Addictive Diseases* (The Haworth Medical Press, an imprint of The Haworth Press, Inc.) Vol. 16, No. 2, 1997, pp. 1-14; and: *Intensive Outpatient Treatment for the Addictions* (ed: Edward Gottheil, and Barry Stimmel) The Haworth Medical Press, an imprint of The Haworth Press, Inc., 1997, pp. 1-14. Single or multiple copies of this article are available for a fee from The Haworth Document Delivery Service [1-800-342-9678, 9:00 a.m. - 5:00 p.m. (EST). E-mail address: getinfo@haworth.com].

tended self-help meetings or continued in outpatient treatment, more often to have been admitted for inpatient treatment or been in jail, less often returned to school and were more often using cocaine.

Clearly, clinicians and researchers need a better understanding of these patients who account for significant attrition, have distinguishing characteristics, and do much more poorly than those who remain in treatment. *[Article copies available for a fee from The Haworth Document Delivery Service: 1-800-342-9678. E-mail address: getinfo@haworth.com]*

INTRODUCTION

A continuing and vexing problem for clinician and researcher alike has been the high rate of dropouts from outpatient substance abuse treatment programs.[1-6] This has led to many studies attempting to identify predictive correlates of attrition/retention. Unfortunately, the results of these studies have been generally weak and inconsistent.[1,3,5-12] What seemed most consistent to Craig,[8] for example, was the inconsistency of the predictors from one study to the next. One of the possible reasons for this inconsistency is that patients drop out for different reasons at different stages of treatment so that variables associated with program dropout would vary with the stage of treatment under study.[13,14]

Baekeland and Lundwall,[1] in their extensive review of the literature on dropouts, had also commented on the different time frames employed in the studies. They recommended a classification into immediate dropout (after 1 visit), rapid dropout (after 1 month) and slow dropout (between 2 and 6 months). More recently, attrition at seven points or stages was described by Howard, Cox, and Saunders.[13] The first three points at which dropout may occur, i.e., before entering the facility, at intake, and during initial screening are included in "preinclusion attrition." After assignment to a treatment (independent variable) is the fourth point and is referred to as "independent-variable attrition." The last three points or stages, i.e., during treatment, at completion of treatment, and at follow-up are included in "postinclusion attrition."

Given the interest in studies of treatment outcome and effectiveness, it is not surprising that most analyses of attrition/retention have focused on postinclusion data of patients who have entered treatments. In this regard, judgments, which may vary, are required regarding what constitutes a suitable and sufficient exposure to a treatment (i.e., how many treatment visits, how much time) in order to be able reasonably to compare the effectiveness of that treatment with other treatments or control conditions.[14] There has been much less emphasis on preinclusion attrition even though studies show that of individuals calling up and making appointments, 50% to 64% fail to show up for an initial appointment.[6,15] Of those keeping their appointment, there are additional significant pretreatment (also referred to as immediate, early, or short-term) attrition losses. Several studies report that 29% to 42% attend one or two intake sessions but do not return for any treatment sessions.[3,5,16,17]

The results of the few available studies of early, pretreatment dropouts from outpatient substance abuse treatment are also weak and inconsistent even though based on the same stage of attrition. Leigh, Ogborne, and Cleland,[3] for example, using regression analysis, found only two of a wide variety of sociodemographic, personality, symptom, treatment history, medical status, and treatment system variables that discriminated between patients who dropped out after one or two sessions in an alcoholism outpatient treatment program and those who satisfactorily completed treatment. These were a social stability score and the absence of dependents at home. Stark and Campbell[5] compared immediate dropouts (after 1 visit) from a substance abuse-treatment program with patients remaining in treatment for at least two months. No major differences were found attributable to demographic or drug use variables except that nonvoluntary (court mandated) patients were more likely to return after the first visit. Regarding personality variables, remainers generally were found to have higher scores on the Millon Clinical Multiaxial Inventory (MCMI) scales indicating more disturbance on scales such as psychotic thinking, psychotic delusions, and paranoia. On the other hand there was an interaction in that amphetamine abusers indicating greater subjective distress on these scales tended to drop out immediately. No differences were found between the groups on the SCL 90. In a study by Kleinman et al.,[16] none of a large battery of variables was found to significantly differentiate cocaine abusers who attended one or two research sessions only, from those returning for one or more therapy sessions.

It should be noted that while these studies focused on early, pretreatment attrition, they differed with respect to (a) drugs of addiction and (b) time in treatment of the comparison groups of patients (i.e., at least one therapy visit, two months of treatment, or treatment completers). Moreover, none of the studies compared these groups at follow-up. The purpose of the present study was to compare the characteristics of one diagnostic group of substance use patients (i.e., cocaine dependence) who dropped out during intake and prior to receiving one outpatient treatment service with those who returned for at least one therapy visit and those who remained for two months or more, and to compare outcomes of these groups at follow-up, nine months after their initial visit.

METHODS

Subjects

Volunteers for a research project to compare the effectiveness of three outpatient drug abuse treatment approaches were recruited from those individuals entering the Jefferson Outpatient Cocaine Treatment Clinic[18] who met the following criteria: first admissions, above the age of 18 years, DSM-III-R diagnosis of cocaine dependence, not overtly psychotic, actively suicidal, or so cognitively impaired as to be unable to participate in the program.

On their first visit to our clinic, patients (regular or research) are registered, receive a handout of program rules and regulations, and complete a set of intake forms, interviews, and questionnaires (i.e., initial assessments). They also meet a counselor who welcomes them, listens to their reasons for seeking admission, and responds to their questions. At some time during the initial session the counselor covers a number of specific issues: (1) the nature of the program, it's three month duration, scheduled weekly urinalyses, and the importance of committing oneself to complete the three month treatment period; (2) rating the relative importance of their individual problems and objectives and the development of an appropriate treatment plan; (3) the significance of HIV testing and counseling; (4) monthly reviews of treatment plans and accomplishments and an end-of-program aftercare plan; and (5) the follow-up process including requests for names, addresses, and phone numbers of two individuals who would likely know of their whereabouts for purposes of follow-up. For those eligible to enter the clinical trial, a description of the research study is presented along with a request to volunteer and sign an informed consent.

On their second visit, all patients (regular or research) complete a detailed psychosocial history data base, attend an AIDS instructional session and meet their therapist. The AIDS instructional module consists of current HIV/AIDS information, a video to reinforce the information, and a discussion of the materials. The therapist discusses the patient's treatment plan, presents an orientation to the program and arranges the next appointment.

Initial Assessments

The information obtained is used for treatment planning, meeting state requirements, record keeping, and data reporting. The set of forms and measures includes: (1) brief intake form covering basic demographic data, previous treatment and employment histories, and personal and family history of substance use; (2) self-administered Milcom[19] personal and family medical history and review of systems; (3) urine drug screen; (4) assessment of cocaine dependence indicating how many of the nine DSM-III-R criteria are present; (5) Addiction Severity Index (ASI),[20,21] a standard instrument of demonstrated reliability and validity indicating difficulties in seven problem areas; (6) Beck Depression Inventory (BDI),[22] a standard, quick measure of depression; (7) Symptom Checklist (SCL-90-R),[23] a quick, multifactor measure of global psychopathology.

Administration of the above battery usually requires one and one-half to one and three-quarter hours but may occasionally take two hours. On the second visit, a detailed, self-administered Psychosocial History Form which includes family, educational, sexual, marital, recreational, vocational, legal, financial management, and drug and alcohol sections is administered which takes about 50 minutes to complete.

Follow-Up

Agreement to be followed up nine months after admission was sought at intake and updated at the end of the treatment period.

Only subjects who agreed to follow-up were contacted. Follow-up interviews were conducted independently by an external contractor. Payment of $20.00 was made for cooperation with the follow-up interview. Measures obtained included: ASI, self-help group attendance (CA, NA, AA), incarceration, treatment, employment.

RESULTS

Of the 447 volunteers for the 3-month treatment study, 123 (27.5%) did not return following intake for even one treatment visit (TV-0). The characteristics of these pretreatment dropouts (TV-0) were compared with the 324 who returned to attend at least one therapy session (TV-1) and with the 118 of these who remained in the program for two months (TV-2M) or more. Of the 324 who received at least one treatment visit, 36.4% remained in treatment for at least two months and 23.8% completed the program.

TV-0 vs. TV-1

At intake, TV-0 individuals, as compared to TV-1s, were significantly less often employed, reported fewer months of employment during the last two years, and more often had cocaine positive urinalyses (Table 1). A smaller proportion of the TV-0 group reported using other drugs in addition to cocaine. On the ASI, TV-0s had less severe medical problems and on the SCL-90 lower scores on the interpersonal sensitivity scale and a tendency for lower scores on the obsessive-compulsive scale than TV-1s.

Since no hypotheses with respect to differences in intake characteristics between the groups were proposed, two-tailed tests of significance were used for the comparisons in Table 1. Regarding follow-up results, however, we expected better outcomes for individuals receiving more treatment and one-tailed tests of significance were used in Table 2.

At 9-month follow-up, individuals who had dropped out without treatment were using cocaine more frequently and were less involved in self-help treatment groups than those who had remained for one or more therapy sessions (Table 2).

TABLE 1. Comparison between 123 patients not attending at least one treatment service and (A) those receiving at least one service, and (B) those receiving at least 8 weeks of treatment:-Intake variables.[a]

	No-Services		At Least One Service		At Least 8 Weeks Tx.	
	N	Mean	N	Mean	N	Mean
DEMOGRAPHICS						
Age at intake	123	31.4	324	32.0	118	31.9
Grade	123	11.3	324	11.5	118	11.5
Mos. emp./24	123	4.1	323	6.6***	118	7.2***
Weekly legal inc.	122	62.5	322	68.8	118	79.2
# Prior tx. D/A	120	.9	322	1.1	118	1.0
Age 1st coc. use	122	24.7	324	24.9	118	24.8
# DSM criteria	79	7.3	270	7.2	95	7.4
ASI PROBLEM SEVERITY						
# Days coc./30	57	8.6	309	7.6	117	6.2
Medical	56	1.5	303	2.5**	114	2.6***
Employment	56	4.3	302	4.1	114	4.0
Alcohol	56	3.3	302	3.9	114	4.2*
Drug	56	6.2	302	6.3	114	6.4
Legal	56	1.6	301	1.6	114	1.8
Fam./Social	56	3.8	302	3.7	113	3.8
Psychological	56	3.3	302	3.4	113	3.4
# Days cont. env./30	59	5.5	309	4.3	116	5.9
PERSONALITY						
Beck Dep Inv.	116	15.9	317	16.0	116	14.2
SCL: Som.	113	53.3	312	54.6	115	54.6
SCL: O/C	113	57.3	312	60.0*	115	60.3**
SCL: Int. sens.	113	59.1	312	62.3**	115	62.5**
SCL: Dep.	113	61.4	312	62.9	115	63.4
SCL: Anx.	113	56.3	312	58.7	115	59.3*
SCL: Hos.	113	57.3	312	56.7	115	57.2
SCL: Ph. anx.	113	57.4	312	59.3	115	60.1**
SCL: Par. ideation	113	60.2	312	61.0	115	60.7
SCL: Psych.	113	61.4	312	63.6	115	64.6**

TABLE 1 (continued)

DEMOGRAPHICS

	No-Services	At Least One Service	At Least 8 Weeks Tx
N=	123	324	118
	%	%	%
Male	59.3	62.0	62.7
African-Am.	91.9	94.1	89.0
Never marr.	78.0	74.7	72.9
Living w. fam.	35.8	35.8	31.4
Caring for dep.	19.5	19.1	16.9
Student	1.6	1.5	1.7
Currently employed	4.9	11.1**	12.7**
Any prev. tx. D/A	45.8	39.1	35.6

CRIMINAL HISTORY

1 or more felony arrests	8.9	16.1	16.9*
1 or more misd. arrests	19.5	13.9	18.6

ROUTE OF COCAINE ADMINISTRATION

% Smoking Cocaine	87.8	88.3	85.6
% IV use	1.6	4.0	5.1
% Snort	10.6	7.7	9.3

SECOND DRUG OF ABUSE

Any 2nd Drug	51.2	62.3**	62.7*

SECOND DRUG OF ABUSE (if any)[b]

N=	63	202	74
Alcohol	76.2	77.7	86.5
Opiates	3.2	5.9	4.1
Marijuana	19.0	14.4	6.8*

URINALYSES

N=	110	295	111
Cocaine+	60.0	48.5**	36.0***
Other Drug+	9.1	8.5	8.1

[a]Differences between columns 1 and 2 and 1 and 3 are tested by t-tests for continuous variables and X^2 for non-continuous variables.
[b]Columns do not sum to 100% as a result of 6 cases reporting the use of miscellaneous drugs (i.e., barbiturates) not having been included.
* $p < .10$.
** $p < .05$.
*** $p < .01$.

TABLE 2. Comparison between patients not attending at least one treatment service and (A) those receiving at least one service, and (B) those receiving at least 8 weeks of treatment:-Follow-up variables.[a]

	No-Services		At Least One Service		At Least 8 Weeks Tx.	
	N	Mean	N	Mean	N	Mean
ASI						
# Days coc./30	34	4.97	228	2.81*	93	1.47**
Medical	34	.13	222	.15	91	.16
Employment	32	.80	214	.85	89	.78
Alcohol	33	.08	219	.11	92	.07
Drug	34	.10	219	.08	90	.06*
Legal	32	.07	210	.04	89	.03
Fam./Social	33	.17	222	.14	91	.16
Psychological	34	.24	219	.21	90	.17*
Days cont. env./30	35	2.89	228	2.03	92	2.00
Categorical Variables:						
N=	123		324		118	
	%		%		%	
Follow-up	64.2		73.1		79.7*	
Inpat. tx.	17.7		13.1		7.4*	
Outpat. tx.	12.7		17.7		27.7*	
Self-help 1 × /wk.	32.9		51.5*		66.0***	
Jail	17.7		12.2		6.4*	
Job	44.3		46.0		50.0	
School	11.4		19.9		29.0**	
Urinalysis:						
Submitted Urine N=	52		161		67	
Cocaine+	59.6		47.2		32.8**	
Other drug+	7.8		6.2		7.5	

[a]Differences between columns 1 and 2 and 1 and 3 are tested by ANCOVA for continuous variables and chi-square for non-continuous variables. One-tailed tests.

* $p < .05$.

** $p < .01$.

*** $p < .001$.

TV-0 vs. TV-2M

Since the TV-1 group included a number of patients who dropped out after only minimal treatment exposure and who might closely resemble the TV-0 group, we compared the pretreatment dropout group with a group of patients who remained in the program for more of a treatment experience. The two month period was chosen to be comparable to the Stark and Campbell[5] study and it so happened that the number of patients remaining for 2 months or more was rather similar to the number who dropped out before attending any therapy sessions.

Actually, the differences between TV-0 and TV-2M were similar to those between TV-0 and TV-1 but stronger. The TV-2M patients, at intake, were significantly more often currently employed, reported more months of employment during the last two years, and less often had cocaine positive urinalyses (Table 1). A larger proportion used other drugs in addition to cocaine and reported one or more felony arrests. On the ASI, the TV-2Ms had more severe medical complaints and tended to have more severe alcohol problems while on the SCL-90 they received significantly higher scores on the interpersonal sensitivity, obsessive-compulsive, phobic anxiety, and psychoticism scales and tended to have higher scores on the anxiety scale than the TV-0s.

At 9-month follow-up, the pretreatment dropouts were doing much less well than those patients who had received at least two months of treatment (Table 2). They were using cocaine more frequently and a larger proportion had urinalyses positive for cocaine than the TV-2Ms. On the ASI, the TV-0s had higher scores on drug problems and psychological problems. More TV-0s had been admitted for inpatient treatment and fewer had entered outpatient treatment or became involved in self-help treatment groups. The TV-0s had more often been in jail and less often returned to school than the TV-2Ms. It should be noted that the above significant differences are probably conservative underestimates since the successful follow-up rate for the TV-0s was much lower than for the TV-2Ms.

DISCUSSION

Of 447 individuals who entered an intensive cocaine outpatient treatment clinic and volunteered during the intake process for a clinical trial, 27.5% dropped out without keeping at least one appointment for a treatment visit. In contrast to the study by Kleinman et al.,[16] we did find differences between the individuals who dropped out without receiving any therapy and those who returned for one or more therapy sessions. The pretreatment dropouts reported a more unstable employment history and were more often recent users of cocaine as indicated by positive admission urinalysis. They also had less severe medical problems and tended to be less interpersonally sensitive and less compulsive than those returning for treatment.

When the pretreatment dropouts were compared with patients who remained in the program for at least two months, the differences were similar to those described above but were more pronounced especially on the psychopathology scales of the SCL-90. Stark and Campbell[5] also reported that patients who remained in treatment for two months or more were more disturbed psychologically than pretreatment dropouts. Interestingly, however, the personality differences they found were on the scales of the MCMI and not on the SCL-90.

To better understand why people enter, remain in, or leave treatment we need to examine preinclusion as well as postinclusion attrition.[13,14] Preinclusion attrition accounts for significantly greater losses of patients from treatment studies and, of course, from treatment, which is unfortunate when we consider the poor outcome results of the pretreatment dropouts. We are unable to claim that our particular treatment was responsible for the better results of the patients who remained in treatment since the patients were not randomly assigned to treatment and no treatment groups. What we are able to state, however, is that the dropouts, for whatever reasons, did very poorly as compared to those who remained in the program. It would seem important, then, to study ways of decreasing preinclusion attrition.

In a previous paper, for example, we reported that of 520 persons who called the clinic for appointments, 188 or 36% arrived for their intake interview. Even though 94% of the appointments were scheduled within six days, we found that the sooner the appointment the greater the likelihood it would be kept. For same day appointments, 60% came in and this percentage decreased significantly to 30% at 6 days.[15] We then attempted to phone the 324 persons (62%) who failed to present for intake and had not called to cancel. We were able to reach 144 (44%) of them and reschedule an appointment for 106 (74%). Of these 106, 49 (46%) kept their intake appointment increasing the overall proportion of callers entering treatment from 188 (36%) to 237 (46%). The question remained, however, as to whether the time and energy expended in outreach efforts would be worth it or might merely result in enrolling poorly motivated patients who would not likely do well. Accordingly, we compared the 188 who kept their initial appointment, the 49 who came in for rescheduled appointments, and a group of 39 patients who walked into the clinic without calling, with respect to early dropping out and retention in treatment. There were no differences among these three groups in 1-day dropouts, 4 week retention, 8 week retention, or treatment completers.[24]

Focusing on aspects of preinclusion attrition has seemed to us to be worthwhile. We found that with minimal programmatic effort, i.e., scheduling appointments "as soon as possible" and calling to reschedule individuals who failed to keep their intake appointments, many individuals came into the clinic who otherwise might have been lost to treatment. Moreover, they were no more likely to drop-out prematurely and were as likely to complete as presumably "better motivated" patients who kept their initial appointment or who were "walk-ins." It seems reasonable to us to recommend further study of the significant numbers of patients who enter treatment and drop out during or after intake without attending therapy and to try and develop techniques to engage such individuals since those distinguishing characteristics (such as, poor work histories, less emotional and physical distress, etc.) which make them identifiable at intake also may lead them to do so much more poorly than those who remain in treatment.

REFERENCES

1. Baekeland F, Lundwall L. Dropping out of treatment: a critical review. Psychol Rev. 1975; 82: 738-783.

2. Fiester AR, Rudestam KE. A multivariate analysis of the early dropout process. J Consult Clin Psychol. 1975; 43: 528-535.

3. Leigh G, Ogburne AC, Cleland P. Factors associated with patient dropout from an outpatient alcoholism treatment service. J Stud Alcohol. 1984; 45: 359-362.

4. Silberfeld M, Glaser FB. Use of the life table method in determining attrition from treatment. J Stud Alcohol. 1978; 39: 1582-1590.

5. Stark MJ, Campbell BK. Personality, drug use, and early attrition from substance abuse treatment. Am J Drug Alcohol Abuse. 1988; 14: 475-485.

6. Stark MJ, Campbell BK, Brinkerhoff CV. "Hello, may we help you?": a study of attrition prevention at the time of the first phone contact with substance-abusing clients. Am J Drug Alcohol Abuse. 1990; 16: 67-76.

7. Craig RJ. Can personality tests predict treatment dropouts? Int J Addict. 1984; 19: 665-674.

8. Craig RJ. Reducing the treatment dropout rate in drug abuse programs. J Subst Abuse Treat. 1985; 2: 209-219.

9. DeLeon G. Therapeutic communities. In: Galanter M, Kleber HD, eds. Textbook of substance abuse treatment. Washington, DC: American Psychiatric Press. 1994: 391-414.

10. Gossop M. Drug dependence: a study of the relationship between motivational, cognitive, social, and historical factors and treatment variables. J Nerv Ment Dis. 1978; 166: 44-50.

11. Hahn J, King KP. Client and environmental correlates of patient attrition from an inpatient alcoholism treatment center. J Drug Educ. 1982; 12: 75-86.

12. Pekarik G, Jones DL, Blodgett C. Personality and demographic characteristics of dropouts and completers in a non-hospital residential alcohol treatment program. Int J Addict. 1986; 21: 131-137.

13. Howard KI, Cox WM, Saunders, SM. Attrition in substance abuse comparative treatment research: the illusion of randomization. In: Onken LS, Blaine JD, eds. Psychotherapy and counseling in the treatment of drug abuse. Washington, DC: NIDA Research Monograph 104, DHHS Publication No. (ADM) 91-1722, 1990: 66-79.

14. Beutler LA. Methodology: what are the design issues involved in the defined research priorities? In: Onken LS, Blaine JD, eds. Psychotherapy and counseling in the treatment of drug abuse. Washington, DC: NIDA Research Monograph 104, DHHS Publication No. (ADM) 91-1722, 1990: 105-118.

15. Fehr BJ, Weinstein SP, Sterling RS, Gottheil E. "As soon as possible:" An initial treatment engagement strategy. Subst Abuse. 1991; 4: 183-189.

16. Kleinman PH, Kang SY, Lipton DS, Woody GE, Kemp J, Millman RB. Retention of cocaine abusers in outpatient psychotherapy. Am J Drug Alcohol Abuse. 1992; 18: 29-43.

17. Gainey RR, Wells EA, Hawkins JD, Catalano RF. Predicting treatment retention among cocaine users. Int J Addict. 1993; 28: 487-505.

18. Weinstein SP, Gottheil E, Sterling RC. Randomized comparison of intensive outpatient vs. individual therapy for cocaine abusers. J Addict. Dis. 1997; 16(2): 41-56.

19. Milcom Systems. Milcom. Libertyville, IL: Milcom Systems, Hollister Inc. 1989.

20. McLellan AT, Luborsky L, O'Brien CP. Improved diagnostic instrument for substance abuse patients: The Addiction Severity Index. J Nerv Ment Dis. 1980; 168: 26-33.

21. McLellan AT, Luborsky L, Cacciola J, Griffith J, Evans F. New data from the Addiction Severity Index: Reliability and validity in three centers. J Nerv Ment Dis. 1985; 173: 412-423.

22. Beck AT. Cognitive therapy and the emotional disorders. New York, NY: International Universities Press. 1976.

23. Shipley WC. Shipley-Institute of Living Scale for measuring intellectual impairment. Hartford, CT: Institute of Living. 1946.

24. Gottheil E, Sterling RC, Weinstein SP. Outreach engagement efforts: are they worth the effort? Am J Drug Alcohol Abuse (In Press).

Efficacy
of Outpatient Intensive Treatment
for Drug Abuse

Jan Campbell, MD
William Gabrielli, MD, PhD
Louise J. Laster, BA
Barry I. Liskow, MD

SUMMARY. Objective: Outpatient intensive treatment for drug and alcohol abuse has become an alternative approach to management of substance abuse. We evaluated the efficacy of an outpatient intensive treatment program for crack cocaine; and the impact of psychiatric diagnosis on outcome variables.

Method: Subjects participating in an outpatient intensive treatment program underwent descriptive testing at entry and at six-month followup. Outcome variables included Addiction Severity Index composite scores and retention in treatment.

Results: Subjects demonstrated significant improvement in ASI scales, over time, with an interaction effect of time and scale. Minimal interaction of psychiatric diagnosis and outcome was found.

Conclusion: Outpatient intensive treatment demonstrated effica-

Jan Campbell, William Gabrielli, Louise J. Laster, and Barry I. Liskow are affiliated with the Psychiatry Service, Kansas City Veterans Affairs Medical Center and Department of Psychiatry, University of Kansas Medical Center.

Address correspondence to: Jan Campbell, MD, Psychiatry Service, VAMC, 4801 Linwood, Kansas City, MO 64128.

Supported by National Institute on Drug Abuse grant DA06954.

[Haworth co-indexing entry note]: "Efficacy of Outpatient Intensive Treatment for Drug Abuse." Campbell, Jan et al. Co-published simultaneously in *Journal of Addictive Diseases* (The Haworth Medical Press, an imprint of The Haworth Press, Inc.) Vol. 16, No. 2, 1997, pp. 15-25; and: *Intensive Outpatient Treatment for the Addictions* (ed: Edward Gottheil, and Barry Stimmel) The Haworth Medical Press, an imprint of The Haworth Press, Inc., 1997, pp. 15-25. Single or multiple copies of this article are available for a fee from The Haworth Document Delivery Service [1-800-342-9678, 9:00 a.m. - 5:00 p.m. (EST). E-mail address: getinfo@haworth.com].

15

cy in reduction of ASI composite scores. Comparison with standard outpatient treatment and inpatient treatment is needed. *[Article copies available for a fee from The Haworth Document Delivery Service: 1-800-342-9678. E-mail address: getinfo@haworth.com]*

INTRODUCTION

The evolution of treatment programs for drug dependence, especially crack cocaine dependence, has been influenced by the large numbers of patients requesting treatment, and by growing concern that the traditional inpatient model may be too costly to apply to a large population, and unnecessary to achieve abstinence. One proposed solution, outpatient intensive treatment, provides frequent contact with patients, psychoeducational programming similar to inpatient treatment, and management of relapse issues in the realistic outpatient setting. We evaluated outcome of treatment in an outpatient intensive program, and here report initial findings of retention in treatment and change in Addiction Severity Index scores in groups of patients with crack cocaine abuse and various associated psychiatric diagnoses.

METHOD

Program Design

The intensive outpatient treatment program was designed to include elements usually found in local treatment programs, in order to improve generalization of findings. Program activities occurred on Monday, Wednesday and Friday, either from 1:00-4:00 pm or from 6:00-9:00 pm. Dinner was offered at 5:00 pm. Each patient had an individual counseling session on Tuesday or Thursday, and those who had families willing to participate were offered family counseling on Tuesday or Thursday. Attendance at community support groups, including Cocaine Anonymous, Narcotics Anonymous, and others, were strongly encouraged. Urine toxicology for illicit drugs was obtained on a random schedule at least weekly and at any time there was suspicion of use of drugs.

The program was structured in three phases, varying in both intensity of contact with treatment staff and in the issues addressed. In Phase I, patients were to attend three-hour segments, three times weekly, with one hour of individual counseling, for a total of 36 hours of group and 4 hours of individual treatment activities. It was therefore possible to complete Phase I attendance requirements in four weeks. Graduation to Phase II required drug-free urine toxicology for four consecutive weeks, a standard that proved difficult for patients to attain. In Phase II, patients were expected to attend at least three hours of group activity weekly and one hour of individual counseling. Patients were expected to continue drug-free toxicology; relapse, as indicated by positive urine sample or self-report, was addressed as an opportunity to learn new coping skills. If relapse extended over several weeks, patients were returned to Phase I intensity of contact. Graduation to Phase III required meeting attendance requirements of 12 hours of group and 4 hours of individual treatment activity, and maintaining drug-free urine toxicology. Phase III treatment activities involved one hour weekly of group or individual treatment, and continuing drug-free urine toxicology.

The initial assessment included an individual interview with a counselor, explanation of the treatment program, and an opportunity to join an on-going group that day or evening. Patients were then scheduled for either afternoon or evening segment attendance, an appointment was made to complete the assessment profile within 7 to 10 days, and a schedule of individual meetings with a counselor was provided.

The content of the Phase I treatment program focused on detoxification, stabilization, and management of any crisis associated with presentation for treatment. Because more than half of the patients came with legal issues including probation and parole referrals and thus were not voluntarily involved in recovery, this phase was marked by struggles with authority and denial. Both supportive and confrontational group activities were used extensively, as well as educational groups regarding physical and emotional effects of crack cocaine and other drug use. Separate group activities for women focused on sexual and reproductive issues. All program participants were given instruction on HIV/AIDS and safe sex practices, especially regarding crack cocaine-related sexual activities in crack houses or with other users. Participants were taught the role of triggers and cues and strategies for avoiding high-risk situations. An introduction to Cocaine Anonymous and Narcotics Anonymous 12-step programs was arranged and patients were encouraged to utilize these and other community support groups.

In Phase II, patients began intensive relapse prevention activities, including developing a map of previous relapse episodes with identification of subtle high-risk situations and apparently unrelated decisions; and self-monitoring activities involving family members or friends able to identify behavioral changes associated with resumption of drug use. Participation in community support or 12-step programs was expected. Information about emergence of psychological issues and psychiatric symptomatology was provided and if indicated, patients were encouraged to obtain further evaluation with the local mental health center staff.

In Phase III, patients continued working with relapse prevention techniques and focused on resolving personal, relationship, employment and legal problems associated with drug use. During this phase, patients might also begin to act as mentors for other patients in Phase I.

Subjects

Subjects were drawn from patients participating in the outpatient treatment program at a community mental health center, described previously. All subjects met DSM-III-R criteria for cocaine dependence; dependence on other drugs was allowed but patients on methadone maintenance were excluded. Patients with psychosis or major medical disorders were not included in this treatment program or research protocol.

At the time of the initial assessment for entry to the treatment program, patients were told about the research protocol involving a comparison of desipramine, carbamazepine and placebo, and were given an opportunity to volunteer. The pharmacotherapy protocol was provided in addition to the core treatment program, and patients who preferred not to participate in the research were encouraged to attend the treatment activities. Those patients who chose the research protocol signed an informed consent allowing administration of a psychological testing battery including the Psychiatric

Diagnostic Interview (PDI),[1] a structured psychiatric interview producing DSM-III-R diagnoses; Addiction Severity Index (ASI);[2] Beck Depression and Beck Anxiety Inventories;[3,4] Halikas-Crosby Drug Impairment Rating Scale for Cocaine (HALDIRS);[5] and NEO,[6] a temperament survey. Subjects also signed informed consent allowing the performance of a physical exam, electrocardiogram, blood chemistries, complete blood count and differential, urinalysis, and urine toxicology. If the results of these evaluations were acceptable, subjects signed informed consent to participate in the pharmacotherapy protocol and were then randomized to active medication or placebo status. During the time period awaiting randomization, subjects attended treatment program activities.

There were 151 subjects in the sample, 105 males and 46 females. The population was predominantly African-American. The mean age for males was 34 and for females was 32.

DATA ANALYSIS

Analysis of variance was used to compare subjects receiving carbamezapine, desipramine or placebo on variables including retention in treatment, days of treatment exposure, drug-free urine toxicology, and ASI composite scores. There were no differences among the drug groups on any of these variables. Results of this analysis have been reported elsewhere.[7] In the following analyses, the three groups were combined.

Analysis of variance for repeated measures and paired t-test for correlated means were used to compare subject scores on the ASI at program entry and at 6 month follow-up across diagnostic categories to determine if significant change occurred, and if there was an interaction between diagnosis and change in ASI scores. Survival analysis was used to compare diagnostic groups on the variable of retention in treatment over a 26-week period. Two analyses were performed. First, all subjects with no diagnosis other than drug dependence or drug and alcohol dependence, diagnosis of depression, antisocial personality disorder, or anxiety disorder were compared; second, subjects were assigned in an hierarchical decision to either depression, antisocial personality disorder, or no psychiatric diagnosis other than drug dependence or drug and alcohol dependence, in that order.

RESULTS

Table 1 displays the frequency and percent of subjects within each psychiatric diagnostic category on the PDI. Subjects meeting criteria for schizophrenia (two) were not clinically ill or receiving treatment for schizophrenia. Subjects with the following diagnoses were included in the data analysis: drug dependence or drug and alcohol dependence only, depression, antisocial personality, and anxiety disorder (including panic). There were 151 subjects, of which 8 were excluded because of incomplete PDIs. Of the remaining 143 subjects, 36 had only drug or drug and alcohol diagnoses; the remainder had at least one psychiatric diagnosis and 57 had two or more diagnoses.

Survival analysis was performed for both hierarchical and non-hierarchical grouping. For the hierarchical grouping, psychiatric diagnosis had no effect on retention in treatment (Chi-square = 1.59, p > .45). In the non-hierarchical analysis, comparing the no-

TABLE 1. Frequency of Psychiatric Diagnoses (N = 143)*

Diagnosis	Frequency	Percent
Drug Dep.	143	100
Alcoholism	61	42.7
Depression	43	30.1
Mania	9	6.3
Schizophrenia	2	1.4
ASP	56	39.2
Anorexia	1	0.7
Bulimia	2	1.4
PTSD	7	4.9
OCD	1	0.7
Phobia	9	6.3
Panic	2	1.4
Gen. Anxiety	9	6.3

*Eight individuals had incomplete or missing P.D.I.s, and were excluded from this analysis. Additionally, of the 143 individuals, 5 met criteria for mental retardation, but these were not found to be clinically relevant.

diagnosis group to all other groups (depression, anxiety and antisocial), the Chi-square = 2.04, p > .15; comparing the no-diagnosis group to the depression group, Chi-square = .02, p > .88; comparing the no-diagnosis group to the antisocial group, Chi-square = 1.24, p > .27; and comparing the no-diagnosis group to the anxiety group, Chi-square = 8.05, p < .005. Figure 1 displays the survival curves for the non-hierarchical groups.

ASI composite scores at entry and six-month follow-up were available for 78 subjects. In a multivariate analysis with individual composite scores as repeated measures over time, highly significant improvement was noted (f (1/75) = 25.27, p < 0.0001), in ASI composite scores regardless of psychiatric diagnosis. In addition, an interaction effect was found between ASI composite scores on each scale and time (f (6/70) = 14.95, p < 0.0001). Reduction in ASI composite scores on each scale using paired t-test for correlated means is displayed in Table 2. Significant reduction in scores was found on the following scales: drug use (t = 7.464, p < 0.0001), legal status (t = 2.973, p < 0.0039), family/social relationships (t = 5.029, p < 0.0001) and psychiatric (t = 4.494, p < 0.0001). A trend to significant improvement was present for the medical status scale (t = 1.82, p < 0.0728). Two scales did not demonstrate significant improvement: alcohol use (t = 1.596, p < 0.1146); and employment status (t = 0.665, p < 0.5081).

FIGURE 1. Subject Retention by Co-Morbid Status

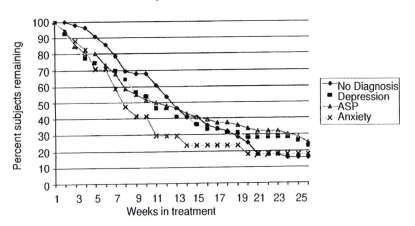

In order to evaluate the impact of psychiatric diagnosis on change in ASI scores, subjects were classified in two ways. First, subjects were classified according to presence of the following diagnoses: depression, anxiety, antisocial personality or no diagnosis other than drug or alcohol and drug dependence. The effect of each diagnosis on ASI scores was then subjected to analysis of variance (see Figure 2 and Table 3). Subjects with depression had a trend toward greater improvement on the medical composite score ($f = 3.41$, $p < 0.0687$) but otherwise did not differ from non-de-

TABLE 2. Mean Improvement in ASI Scores from Baseline to 6-Month Follow-Up, Paired T-Test for Correlated Means

	Mean (SD)	T	prob
Medical	.056 (.273)	1.82	.0728
Employment	−.062 (.827)	−0.665	.5081
Alcohol	.037 (.204)	1.596	.1146
Drug	.082 (.097)	7.464	.0001
Legal	.094 (.281)	2.973	.0039
Family/Social	.134 (.235)	5.029	.0001
Psychiatric	.103 (.2)	4.494	.0001

FIGURE 2. Mean ASI Change Scores by Co-Morbid Group

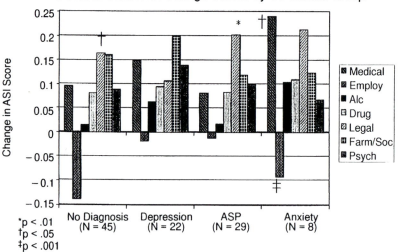

TABLE 3. ASI Change Scores by Co-Morbid Group Mean and Standard Deviations

	No Diagnosis	Depression	Antisocial	Anxiety
Medical	.095 (.29)	.148 (.29)	.081 (.30)	.240 (.30)
Employment	−.139 (1.05)	.018 (.21)	−.031 (.31)	−.927 (2.36)
Alcohol	.014 (.19)	.062 (.19)	.016 (.16)	.104 (.25)
Drug	.081 (.09)	.094 (.08)	.082 (.09)	.109 (.06)
Legal	.164 (.27)	.106 (.27)	.202 (.26)	.213 (.29)
Fam/Social	.160 (.22)	.196 (.26)	.119 (.17)	.124 (.23)
Psychiatric	.088 (.18)	.139 (.24)	.099 (.20)	.067 (.07)

pressed subjects. Antisocial subjects demonstrated significant improvement on the legal composite score (f = 6.00, p < 0.0166) but did not differ from non-antisocial subjects on any other score. Subjects with anxiety had significant improvement on the medical composite score (f = 4.05, p < 0.0479) but on the employment scale, had significant decline in score (f = 11.03, p < 0.0014). Anxious subjects did not differ from non-anxious subjects on any other ASI composite score. Subjects with no diagnosis other than drug or drug and alcohol dependence demonstrated significant improvement on the legal composite score (f = 4.96, p < 0.0290) but otherwise did not differ from subjects with psychiatric diagnoses.

When subjects were classified in an hierarchical model with depression taking precedence over antisocial personality and antisocial personality taking precedence over anxiety, subjects with antisocial personality had significant improvement in legal composite score compared to those with depression or only drug and alcohol dependence (f = 4.69, p < .02). No other differences were found among the three groups (Figure 3).

DISCUSSION

Subjects attending this outpatient intensive treatment program for primarily crack cocaine-dependent patients achieved very significant reductions in ASI scores at 6-month follow-up, supporting

FIGURE 3. Mean ASI Change Scores by Co-Morbid Group (Hierarchical)

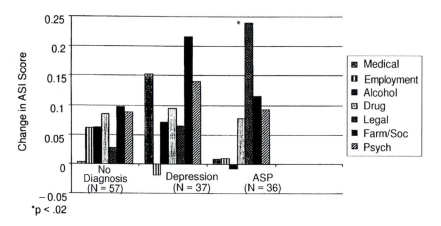

*p < .02

clinical observations that outpatient intensive treatment is effective. It must be noted that the experimental group was not compared to a control group, either an inpatient treatment group, or patients receiving treatment in standard outpatient programs, thus it is unknown whether more improvement could be expected with other treatment modalities. Nevertheless, it is important to recognize the significant personal and social impact of drug and alcohol treatment, reflected in reduction of legal complications and family and social conflict, and psychiatric symptoms on the ASI composite scores.

Subjects with the diagnosis of anxiety were significantly less likely to remain in treatment through the six-month period than were subjects with no diagnosis, depression, or antisocial personality. It is possible that the group setting of treatment and the confrontational approach in some of the discussion groups may have been unacceptable to subjects with anxiety disorders. Although there was a significant improvement in the psychiatric composite scale scores of the entire group of patients from program entry to follow-up, a significant change was not noted for those subjects with diagnoses of depression or anxiety. This minimal interaction between outcome and presence of psychiatric diagnosis was unexpected in light of the clinical impression that "dual-diagnosis" patients are less successful in treatment. This effect may have occurred partly because the ASI does not gather detailed information regarding psychiatric symptoms and treatment received. Other rating scales designed to measure changes in specific psychiatric symptoms and associated behavior at shorter intervals than six months would perhaps be more useful in determining changes in depression and anxiety associated with drug and alcohol treatment.

REFERENCES

1. Othmer E, Penick EC, Powell BJ. Psychiatric Diagnostic Interview-Revised. Western Psychological Services, Los Angeles: 1987.

2. McLellan TA, Luborsky L, Cacciola J, Griffith J, McGahan P, O'Brien CP. Addiction Severity Index. National Institute on Drug Abuse, US Dept. of Health and Human Services. Washington, DC: 1985.

3. Beck AT, Ward CH, Mendelson M. An Inventory for Measuring Depression. Arch Gen Psychiat. 4:561-571, 1961.

4. Beck AT, Steer RA. Beck Anxiety Checklist Manual. Center for Cognitive Therapy, Dept. of Psychiatry, Univ. of Pennsylvania Medical Center, Philadelphia, PA. 1987.

5. Halikas J, Crosby R. Drug Impairment Rating Scale for Cocaine. Dept. of Psychiatry, Univ. of Minnesota, Minneapolis, MN. 1992.

6. Costa P, McCrae R. NEO Personality Inventory. Psychological Assessment Resources, Inc., Odessa, FL. 1985

7. Campbell JL, Thomas HM, Liskow BI, Gabrielli W, Penick EC, Laster L. Effect of carbamezapine and desipramine on treatment retention and urine toxicology in outpatient crack cocaine abusers. New Research Abstracts, American Psychiatric Press, 1995.

Evaluation of a Residential Program Using the Addiction Severity Index and Stages of Change

William G. Campbell, MD

SUMMARY. Fifty six individuals admitted to Recovery Acres (a thirty five bed male residential recovery program/half way house) were evaluated using the Addiction Severity Index (ASI) and Socrates, an instrument designed to measure stage of change. Composite scores obtained from the ASI indicated that major problems were present in the areas of employment, alcohol, family/social, and emotional functioning. Stages of Change revealed 27% to be in preparation, 67% action, and 6% in maintenance.

Patients left Recovery Acres either through relapse, or to follow a non-residential program. Follow-up of 26 cases revealed that residents showed statistically significant improvement in areas of alcohol, drug, family/social and emotional problems. Employment, medical, and legal problems as identified by the ASI composite score were significant indicators of negative outcome. Employment still remained a problem three months after admission for most residents. Stage of Change did not predict outcome in terms of abstinence or residential status. *[Article copies available for a fee from The Haworth Document Delivery Service: 1-800-342-9678. E-mail address: getinfo@haworth.com]*

William G. Campbell is affiliated with the Addiction Centre, Foothills Provincial Hospital, 1403-29 Street N.W., Calgary, Alberta, Canada, T2N 2T9.

[Haworth co-indexing entry note]: "Evaluation of a Residential Program Using the Addiction Severity Index and Stages of Change." Campbell, William G. Co-published simultaneously in *Journal of Addictive Diseases* (The Haworth Medical Press, an imprint of The Haworth Press, Inc.) Vol. 16, No. 2, 1997, pp. 27-39; and: *Intensive Outpatient Treatment for the Addictions* (ed: Edward Gottheil, and Barry Stimmel) The Haworth Medical Press, an imprint of The Haworth Press, Inc., 1997, pp. 27-39. Single or multiple copies of this article are available for a fee from The Haworth Document Delivery Service [1-800-342-9678, 9:00 a.m. - 5:00 p.m. (EST). E-mail address: getinfo@haworth.com].

INTRODUCTION

Recovery Acres in Calgary, Alberta, is a 35 bed male treatment program/half-way house, which has a Mission Statement "to provide an effective program based upon the principles of Alcoholics Anonymous to help alcohol and drug abusers recover." Patients are initially screened by Recovery Acres staff, for suitability to enter the program. They are assessed by a psychologist. They may live in the facility for up to twelve months. The focus of the program is on abstinence; however, patients are also encouraged and expected to find employment after an initial two week mandatory program. Successful patients leave Recovery Acres to live elsewhere and continue an alcohol/drug free life, others return to alcohol/drug use.

Apart from testimony and individual observation, no evidence existed to show the value of Recovery Acres. The evaluation had several purposes: to determine any admission characteristics that would affect outcome, to quantify any changes in life areas of those patients at Recovery Acres, and to determine if the program (both residential and nonresidential) offered by Recovery Acres "worked."* It was hoped this information would allow the Board of Directors to determine the quality and effectiveness of the program and be in a position to determine what changes, if any could or should be instituted. The study used the Addiction Severity Index (ASI)[1] to assess severity of problems in various life areas on admission and to document and quantify any changes seen over a three month interval. As part of the initial assessment, the stage of change for each client was assessed using Socrates, a self-report instrument.[2] It was felt that the stage of change instrument might be used to determine if a potential client of Recovery Acres was ready or in a position to become abstinent.

---

*"The program works." This phase first appeared in Alcoholics Anonymous literature in 1939 when used as the title for the Works Publishing Company which produced The Big Book of Alcoholics Anonymous and means that those who follow the recommended twelve steps can recover from alcohol dependence.

PROCEDURE

The Addiction Severity Index and Socrates were administered to 56 consecutive admissions to Recovery Acres by a single interviewer. Approximately three months later, 26 of the original 56 individuals were reassessed again using the Addiction Severity Index. Results are tabulated against outcomes. Outcomes for those individuals who did not receive a follow-up ASI were obtained from house staff at Recovery Acres and were in concordance with those obtained from the ASI. Outcome was studied according to those who remained alcohol/drug free and those who did not: and of the alcohol/drug free patients, those who stayed at Recovery Acres and those who did not.

RESULTS

Demographics of the patients on admission are shown in Table 1. No significant demographic difference was observed between those who were followed and those who were not ($p > 0.05$). A non-significant difference was noted in the years education of those followed, 12.3 ± 4 compared with those not followed 10.8 ± 2 ($p = 0.08$). Initial ASI composite scores and initial stages of change are shown in Table 2. Table 3 shows initial values for troubled or bothered by, and need for counseling in the seven different life areas as well as how the patients ranked the severity and need for treatment in each category.

A comparison of initial scores between those reported using alcohol/drugs and those reported alcohol/drug free (both in and out of residence) is shown in Table 4. Thirteen individuals were reported using alcohol/drugs at three months while 43 were reported alcohol/drug free, a rate of 77%.

In Table 5, the ASI composite scores for those who, while remaining alcohol/drug free did not remain residents, are compared with those who stayed in residence. Scores with rank for "troubled or bothered by," and "need for counseling" for the two groups, both alcohol/drug free, in and not in residence at three months are seen in Table 6, as well as the ranking of these problems for each group.

TABLE 1. Demographics (N = 56)

Age (years)	34.4 ± 9
Education (years)	11.5 ± 3

Race (%)

Caucasian	93
Metis/Native	5
Asian	2

Religion (%)

Catholic	18
Protestant	9
Islamic	2
Jewish	2
Other	7
None	62

Marital Status (%)

Married/CL	19
Separated/Divorced	32
Never Married	48

Employment Status (%)

Full Time	30
Part Time	4
Unemployed	66

Analysis of the ASI composite scores (initial and three months) was then carried out to determine of those who were alcohol/drug free and followed, what changes, if any, had occurred for nonresidents (Table 7), and residents of Recovery Acres (Table 8).

TABLE 2. Initial ASI Composite Score and Initial Stage of Change (N = 56)

ASI Composite Score

Medical	0.15 ± 0.29
Employment	0.60 ± 0.33
Alcohol	0.56 ± 0.26
Drug	0.15 ± 0.14
Legal	0.11 ± 0.17
Family/social	0.35 ± 0.25
Emotional	0.45 ± 0.21

State of Change

	N (%)
Pre-contemplation	— —
Contemplation	— —
Preparation	14 (27)
Action	34 (67)
Maintenance	3 (6)

DISCUSSION

On admission, patients had minimal stabilizing influences in their lives, the majority were unmarried, unemployed and had a low average education (Table 1). This instability may be a result of an alcohol/drug problem causing poor socialization or it could be hypothesized the poor quality of life in these areas led to alcohol/drug problems.

The admission ASI composite scores (Table 3) are similar to those of other programs for males with significant alcohol/drug problems.[3] Also, the majority of individuals on admission were in the preparation or action state of change with some in the maintenance state. Thus, individuals on admission to Recovery Acres had significant alcohol/drug problems and were in a state compatible with becoming alcohol/drug free.

In the thirty days prior to admission to Recovery Acres, patients

TABLE 3. Initial Values for Troubled in the Past 30 Days, and Importance of Counseling

	Troubled past 30 days (0-4) (N = 56)		Importance of Counseling (0-4) (N = 56)	
	Score	Rank	Score	Rank
Medical	0.7	5	0.5	5
Employment	1.7	4	1.7	4
Alcohol	2.8	3	3.5	1
Drugs	1.7	4	2.2	3
Legal	0.68	6	0.32	6
Family/Social	2.9/1.9	2	2.2/2.0	3
Emotional	3.0	1	3.2	2

reported being most troubled by emotional and family problems while feeling that alcohol and emotional problems were the two areas in which they most required counseling (Table 3). Employment, alcohol and drug problems were rated moderate when scaled on bothered or troubled by, while legal and medical problems were rated lowest. The importance of the family in recovery is often stressed, and while alcoholism is often described as a family disease, this area rated second after emotional problems as causing bother or trouble, and third requiring counseling (after emotional problems and alcohol problems) in the thirty days prior to admission.

When the Initial ASI composite scores of those who have returned to alcohol/drug use at three months are compared to those who remain alcohol/drug free, significant differences are seen in the areas of medical, employment, and legal problems (Table 4). Those who remain alcohol/drug free have significantly lower initial composite scores in these three areas, with the scores for medical and legal problems being 0.1 or less. No significant difference is noted in the areas of alcohol, drug, family/social, or emotional problems. Emotional problems include psychiatric interactions and this lack of difference suggests that for this population, psychiatric co-morbidity did not predict outcome. The most significant change is seen in

TABLE 4. Initial Values of Those Reported Using Alcohol/Drugs and Those Reported Not Using Alcohol/Drugs at Three Months

	Returned to Alcohol/ Drug Use (N = 13)	Alcohol/Drug Free (N = 43)	P
Age	33.5 ± 7.6	34.7 ± 9.4	0.70
Schooling	10.5 ± 2.3	11.7 ± 3.2	0.17
ASI Composite Score			
Medical	0.29 ± 0.40	0.10 ± 0.24	0.05*
Employment	0.78 ± 0.33	0.55 ± 0.24	0.02*
Alcohol	0.54 ± 0.26	0.49 ± 0.26	0.83
Drug	0.15 ± 0.16	0.15 ± 0.11	0.99
Legal	0.18 ± 0.25	0.08 ± 0.14	0.05*
Family/Social	0.35 ± 0.32	0.35 ± 0.27	0.99
Psychological	0.47 ± 0.26	0.46 ± 0.21	0.85
Stage of Change	N (%)	N (%)	
Preparation	3 (25)	11 (31)	
Action	8 (67)	26 (67)	0.91
Maintenance	1 (8)	2 (5)	

the area of employment problems (p = 0.02). The Employment ASI composite score was compared to age, education, and the ASI composite score for legal problems, but no significant difference was found between the ASI composite score and age, education, or ASI composite score for legal problems (p = 0.70, 0.17, and 0.13, respectively).

Since the initial ASI composite score for employment problems was the most significant in determining who would or would not remain alcohol/drug free at three months, even in a supportive environment, such as that at Recovery Acres, the ASI composite score for employment problems was examined. It is composed of four questions;

1. A valid drivers license.
2. An automobile for use.
3. Days paid for working in the past thirty.
4. Amount received for employment in the past thirty days.

While weighted in favor of the availability and use of an automobile, there was no statistical difference between those who did or did not have a valid drivers license ($p = 0.12$) or had an automobile available for use ($p = 0.29$) in the previous thirty days for those who did or did not remain alcohol/drug free. Significant difference was seen between those who did or did not remain alcohol/drug free at three months in the number of days paid for working in the previous

TABLE 5. Initial Values for Those Alcohol/Drug Free Resident and Non-resident

	Nonresident (N = 23)	Resident (N = 15)	P
Age (years)	33.65 ± 8.7	34.20 ± 7.7	0.84
Education (years)	10.91 ± 3.0	11.93 ± 2.02	0.26
ASI Composite Score			
Medical	0.23 ± 0.36	0.00	0.00
Employment	0.61 ± 0.33	0.61 ± 0.31	0.99
Alcohol	0.49 ± 0.30	0.57 ± 0.28	0.38
Drug	0.16 ± 0.13	0.14 ± 0.11	0.55
Legal	0.12 ± 0.20	0.06 ± 0.12	0.29
Family/Social	0.37 ± 0.26	0.30 ± 0.24	0.37
Emotional	0.44 ± 0.22	0.44 ± 0.20	0.92
Stage of Change	N (%)	N (%)	
	(N = 15)	(N = 14)	
Preparation	4 (22)	5 (36)	
Action	11 (48)	7 (43)	.84
Maintenance	1 (4)	2 (14)	

TABLE 6. Severity and Rating of Those Who Were Alcohol/Drug Free and Nonresident and Resident for "Bothered or Troubled By" and "Need for Counseling" (Scale 0-4)

	Nonresident (N = 23) Score/Rank		Resident (N = 15) Score/Rank	
	Troubled/Rank	Need/Rank	Troubled/Rank	Need/Rank
Medical	0.93/6	0.60/6	0.00/7	0.00/7
Employment	1.74/5	1.43/5	1.80/3	2.20/3
Alcohol	2.56/2	3.30/1	2.80/2	3.53/1
Drug	1.96/4	2.43/3	1.60/4	2.13/4
Legal	0.78/7	0.26/7	0.40/6	0.20/6
Family/Social	2.39/3	2.39/4	1.53/5	1.87/5
Emotional	2.96/1	2.95/2	3.00/1	2.30/2

thirty (p = 0.02) and in the amount received for employment in the past thirty days (p = 0.03). These two questions appear to be most significant, in addition to the severity of medical and legal problems, in forecasting who will or will not remain alcohol/drug free at three months.

Stage of change was of no value in forecasting which individuals would or would not remain alcohol/drug free at three months. No statistical difference is seen in the state of change of those individuals who remained abstinent and those who did not (p = 0.91). Stage of change did not differentiate between those alcohol/drug free at three months, who would or would not be a resident (p = 0.81) (Table 5). When the initial ASI composite scores of those who were alcohol/drug free and were or were not residents of Recovery Acres at three months are compared, only the area of medical problems (Table 5) shows significance (p < 0.001). No significant difference was seen in other life areas and this suggests that those with fewer initial medical problems would more likely be residents of Recovery Acres three months later.

Alcohol/drug free residents and nonresidents rated emotional problems as most bothersome or troubling and need for counseling for alcohol problems as primary (Table 4). The two groups differed

TABLE 7. Initial and Three Months ASI Composite Scores for Those Non-residents Followed and Alcohol/Drug Free (N = 8)

	Composite Score		
	Initial	Three Months	P
Medical	0.25 ± 0.34	0.08 ± 0.17	0.11
Employment	0.59 ± 0.28	0.46 ± 0.22	0.10
Alcohol	0.38 ± 0.21	0.13 ± 0.16	0.01*
Drug	0.10 ± 0.12	0.01 ± 0.03	0.14
Legal	0.11 ± 0.17	0.05 ± 0.11	0.14
Family/Social	0.43 ± 0.38	0.32 ± 0.24	0.14
Emotional	0.41 ± 0.28	0.25 ± 0.20	0.08

TABLE 8. Initial and Three Months ASI Composite Scores for Those Both Alcohol/Drug Free and in Residence (N = 14)

	Composite Score		
	Initial	Three Months	P
Medical	0	0	—
Employment	0.62 ± 0.32	0.44 ± 0.27	0.067
Alcohol	0.55 ± 0.26	0.09 ± 0.16	0.000*
Drug	0.17 ± 0.10	0.03 ± 0.06	0.003*
Legal	0.06 ± 0.24	0.15 ± 0.17	0.943
Family/Social	0.31 ± 0.24	0.15 ± 0.17	0.033*
Psychological	0.43 ± 0.21	0.11 ± 0.15	0.003*

in how family/social problems and employment problems were rated. Those who remained in Recovery Acres rated employment problems as the third most severe causing trouble or bother compared to those who did not stay in Recovery Acres who rated employment problems as fifth causing trouble or bother. Those who did not remain in Recovery Acres rated family/social problems as third most severe in causing trouble or bother and fourth in need for counseling compared with those who remained in Recovery Acres who rated family/social problems as fifth in troubled or bothered, and need for counseling. Those that did not remain as residents were more concerned with family problems and perhaps felt that they could not adequately deal with family issues as residents. Those that felt they had more serious employment problems and that family/social problems were less pressing (perhaps loss of family support due to alcohol/drug use?) remained as residents of Recovery Acres.

THREE MONTH FOLLOW-UP

Initial and ASI composite scores of those who were alcohol/drug free and not in residence (Table 7) show that while improvement occurs in all areas, statistical significance is present only in the area of alcohol/drug problems, however the number studied is low, (N = 8). The significant improvement in the alcohol/drug problem and not in other areas suggests that while they are no longer experiencing problems with alcohol these individuals are still experiencing significant problems in other life areas at three months. This nonresident alcohol/drug free group rated "troubled or bothered by family problems" as third most severe. Initial perceived severity of family problems that precluded residence at Recovery Acres would appear to have a negative effect on recovery although improvement does occur in all life areas, apart from the alcohol area, it is not significant. A marked, but not significant improvement, is noted in emotional problems.

More positive significant changes are seen when the initial and three month ASI composite scores are compared for residents of Recovery Acres (Table 8). Statistically significant improvement occurs in the areas of alcohol, drug, family/social, and emotional problems. While the employment ASI Composite Score improves from 0.62 ± 0.32 to $-.44 \pm 0.27$, it is not significant (p = 0.07). These individuals rated "troubled or bothered by" employment problems third alter emotional and alcohol problems on admission (Table 4). They also felt a greater "need for counseling" than those alcohol/drug free but who were nonresidents. Employment problems may have been one of the initial reasons for becoming a resident at Recovery Acres, but even in such a supportive environment, it still remains a problem three months later.

The Medical ASI Composite score is not significant at three months being nil to begin with, this being one of the factors that differed between residents and nonresidents (the others being the reported degree of severity of "troubled or bothered by," and "need for counseling"). The three month Legal ASI composite score is slightly higher but not significant and it is hypothesized that residents that remained alcohol/drug free began to deal with some legal issues that had not been of immediate concern on admission.

Since no focused ongoing therapy for family/social or emotional problems is part of Recovery Acres program, the significant improvement in the family/social and emotional ASI composite scores at three months attests that the initial problems in these areas were alcohol/drug induced as becoming alcohol/drug free without any other focused treatment elicits such positive change.

CONCLUSION

Those patients (both resident and nonresident) attending the program and became alcohol/drug free improved. Becoming alcohol/drug free depended on the severity of initial employment, medical, and legal problems. Remaining in residence, as opposed to leaving the program, depended on the severity of initial medical problems and the degree to which initial employment and family/social problems are rated on the scales; "troubled or bothered by," and "need for counseling." Those with lower medical ASI composite scores, higher perceived employment "troubled or bothered by" and "need for counseling" tended to remain as residents, while those rating family/social "troubles or bothers," and "need for counseling" higher became nonresidents.

The conclusion is that Recovery Acres does "work." However, this study suggests that Recovery Acres' most important role is that of encouraging abstinence using the "twelve steps of Alcoholics Anonymous" and that abstinence is what "works." Although it is well known that alcoholics must be abstinent in order to recover, the study suggests that both initial recovery and continued alcohol/drug abstinence are affected by other variables, the most significant being employment. As well, those individuals that did well had fewer medical, employment, and legal problems on admission. Stage of Change was not found to be a useful assessment instrument to supply information regarding outcome.

The Board of Directors at Recovery Acres recognizes that in order to be comfortable and stable in recovery, an individual must be and act responsible for themselves and that employment is vital in order to achieve this goal. The program of Recovery Acres encourages and expects individuals to find employment after the initial two week day program. Even so, the results show that residents still had significant employment problems after three months of being alcohol/drug free in residence, although the improvement in other areas of their life was impressive.

Although the Program offered by Recovery Acres has been shown to be effective, any program can be improved. Areas in a patients' life that pose difficulty must be identified, addressed and the program then modified in order to address these needs and to help patients achieve and maintain a healthy and alcohol/drug free lifestyle. Changes are being made in the Recovery Acres program to better identify and deal with problem areas in the patients lives.

REFERENCES

1. McLellan AT, Luborsky L, O'Brien CP, Woody LE. An improved evaluation instrument for substance abuse patients; The Addiction Severity Index. J of Nerv Ment Dis. 1980; 168:26-33.

2. Miller WR. Socrates. Unpublished instrument. 1993.

3. McLellan AT, Kushner H, Metzger D, Peters R, Smith I, Grissom G, Pettinati H, and Argeriou M. The Fifth Edition of the Addiction Severity Index: Historical Critique and Normative Data. J Subst. Abuse. Trt. 1992.

Randomized Comparison of Intensive Outpatient vs. Individual Therapy for Cocaine Abusers

Stephen P. Weinstein, PhD
Edward Gottheil, MD, PhD
Robert C. Sterling, PhD

SUMMARY. One of the fastest growing approaches to treating cocaine addiction is intensive outpatient treatment (INT). Nevertheless, there have been no previously reported controlled clinical trials comparing this approach to the more traditional (IND) or individual plus group (IND-GRP). This early report of the results of a clinical trial comparing these three approaches indicated that patients who remained in treatment and completed a twelve-week course of care

---

Stephen P. Weinstein, Edward Gottheil, and Robert C. Sterling are affiliated with the Department of Psychiatry and Human Behavior, Thomas Jefferson University.

Address correspondence to: Stephen P. Weinstein, PhD, Department of Psychiatry and Human Behavior, Jefferson Medical College, 1201 Chestnut Street, 15th Floor, Philadelphia, PA 19107.

This research was supported in part by Grant # 1 R18 DA 06166 from the National Institute on Drug Abuse and performed under the auspices of the Commonwealth Office of Drug and Alcohol Programs and the Philadelphia Department of Public Health, Coordinating Office for Drug and Alcohol Abuse Programs. Its contents are solely the responsibility of the authors and do not necessarily represent the official views of the awarding agencies NIDA, ODAP, and CODAAP.

[Haworth co-indexing entry note]: "Randomized Comparison of Intensive Outpatient vs. Individual Therapy for Cocaine Abusers." Weinstein, Stephen P., Edward Gottheil, and Robert C. Sterling. Co-published simultaneously in *Journal of Addictive Diseases* (The Haworth Medical Press, an imprint of The Haworth Press, Inc.) Vol. 16, No. 2, 1997, pp. 41-56; and: *Intensive Outpatient Treatment for the Addictions* (ed: Edward Gottheil, and Barry Stimmel) The Haworth Medical Press, an imprint of The Haworth Press, Inc., 1997, pp. 41-56. Single or multiple copies of this article are available for a fee from The Haworth Document Delivery Service [1-800-342-9678, 9:00 a.m. - 5:00 p.m. (EST). E-mail address: getinfo@ haworth.com].

demonstrated significant improvements in drug use and psychological functioning. However, INT, IND, and IND-GRP did not differ on any of the assessments made during treatment or at treatment completion. The results underscored the importance of remaining in a course of care in order to effect behavioral change. A next step would involve a systematic comparison of those persons who do best in each modality in an effort to define the variables which could help match a patient to a treatment in which he/she is most likely to remain. *[Article copies available for a fee from The Haworth Document Delivery Service: 1-800-342-9678. E-mail address: getinfo@haworth.com]*

INTRODUCTION

This paper will describe a 5 year study conducted at Thomas Jefferson University in Philadelphia in which we compared a newly designed Intensive Outpatient Treatment (INT) model with our more standard approaches, i.e., outpatient individual therapy (IND) and individual therapy plus a weekly group (IND-GRP) in a controlled comparison, random assignment design.

The research involved having 450 cocaine dependent volunteers assigned on a random basis for a period of three months to individual counseling for one hour weekly (IND), individual counseling plus a group session once weekly (IND-GRP) or the intensive group treatment program (INT). It was hypothesized that patients in INT would show significantly better performance than those in IND-GRP treatment, who would in turn show significantly better performance than those in the IND treatment on the following criteria: (A) retention in treatment; (B) reduction in drug use; (C) decreased psychological symptoms; (D) improvement on self-assessments of problem areas.

BACKGROUND

In the late 1980's the rapid escalation of cocaine abuse, which began in the 1970's and early 1980's, led to a sharp increase in requests for treatment services. By 1988, the cocaine epidemic which previously had not really impacted on the treatment service system,[1-3] finally began to severely stretch the available community resources. The growing national awareness of the devastating consequences of cocaine abuse,[4] and the recognition of an association between substance abuse and HIV infection and heterosexual AIDS[5-7] added to the sense of urgency in the country.

Philadelphia, reflecting the national scene, was also experiencing long waiting lists for services as well as high drop-out rates.[8-9] There was a clear need not only for expanded capacity, but perhaps for new or different services. At that time, our own review of the literature indicated that many new and older psychological and pharmacological treatments were being tried, but no preferred treatment for cocaine dependence had emerged.[1,10-13] A new intensive outpatient treatment approach was being tried, and Washton[14] argued rather cogently for the value of such an approach. While no one of the many treatment techniques that were being tried was found to be especially effective, Intensive Outpatient Treatment did emerge as a new approach which has become increasingly popular.

Within our own outpatient drug free program we too were receiving larger numbers of applications for admission from cocaine and particularly crack cocaine dependent users. We also found that many of these applicants failed to show for their first visit and often did not return after one visit. In an effort to help the city of Philadelphia as well as ourselves cope with the problems of waiting lists and early dropouts, we developed and implemented the Jefferson Intensive Outpatient Cocaine Program in late 1988.

The new program offered a limited 3-month intensive treatment exposure involving group meetings and educational activities for three hours, on three days each week. The aims of this Intensive program model (INT) were to: increase the capacity of the city's service delivery system; maintain a rapid (1 to 3 day), no waiting list admission policy; and focus on attempts to engage patients in therapy and improve retention. Since this was to be a brief 3-month duration program (to enable us to continue to meet the demand for services by admitting new patients) we also planned to refer patients completing their three months with us to other standard outpatient programs for continuing care. The design emphasized the use of limited resources to provide maximal patient care and service impact.

METHODS

Intake

During their first visit to the Intensive Outpatient Cocaine Treatment Clinic, patients are registered, receive a handout of program rules and procedures, complete a set of intake forms, interviews and questionnaires, and meet a counselor. The counselor conducts an intake interview which includes the development of a treatment plan with the patient indicating which of the patient's individual problems are felt to be most important to address along with relevant goals, objectives, and action steps.

The participants for the research project were recruited from among those individuals entering this newly established Intensive Outpatient Cocaine Treatment Clinic. Those asked to volunteer were first admissions, above the age of 18 years, with a DSM-III-R diagnosis of cocaine dependence who were not overtly psychotic, actively suicidal, or so cognitively impaired as to be unable to understand informed consent or to participate in our programming. Those who did volunteer and signed an informed consent were assigned on a random basis to IND, IND-GRP, or INT. All other patients entered the INT program.

Assessments

The information obtained from both research and regular patients includes: (1) brief intake form covering basic demographic data, previous treatment and employment histories, and personal and family history of substance use; (2) self-administered Milcom[15] personal and family medical history and review of systems; (3) urine drug screen utilizing the Bayer Chem-1 Immunoanalyzer at a sensitivity of 300 nanograms per ml; (4) assessment of cocaine dependence indicating how many of the nine DSM-III-R criteria are present; (5) AIDS Knowledge Survey (AKS), a modified version of a form widely used in the city; (6) Addiction Severity Index (ASI), a standard instrument of demonstrated reliability and validity indicating difficulties in seven problem areas;[16,17] (7) Beck Depression Inventory (BDI), a standard, quick measure of depression;[18] (8) Symptom Checklist (SCL-90-R), a quick, multifactor measure of global psychopathology.[19] Administration of the above battery usually requires one and one-half hours but may occasionally take up to two hours.

On the second visit a self-administered Psychosocial History Form which includes family, educational, sexual, marital, recreational, vocational, legal, financial management, and drug and alcohol sections is administered which takes about 50 minutes to complete. Also, after the AIDS educational module is presented, the AKS is administered again. Research volunteers were paid $30.00 for their participation in an additional testing session.

Treatment Evaluation

The treatment plans initiated during the first visit are reviewed and updated monthly. Decrease in drug use, participation in treatment and the degree of improvement for each of the patient's three most important self-identified problems listed on the treatment plan are discussed by patient and therapist and rated on 7-point scales.

At the end of the 12th treatment week, in addition to the treatment plan review, other in-treatment measures such as the number and percentage of scheduled sessions attended (excused absence counted as attendance) and the number and percentage of positives for cocaine and other non-prescribed drugs on weekly drug screens are recorded and totals or means calculated as appropriate. Initial assessments 6,7,8 are repeated.

Follow-Up

Agreement to be followed up nine months after admission was sought at intake and updated at the end of the treatment period. Only subjects who agreed to follow-up were contacted. Follow-up interviews were conducted by an independent contractor. Payment of $20.00 was made for cooperation with the follow-up interview. Measures obtained included: ASI; self-help group attendance (CA, NA, AA); incarceration; treatment; employment.

Treatment Approach

For our individual and group treatments, the therapeutic attitude of our counselors might best be characterized as problem focused, exploratory, supportive, and expressive as needed. Our therapeutic approach is aimed at defined and expected behavioral changes and conducted according to mutually agreed upon treatment plans, and does not adhere to a single, therapeutic model. Rather, as recommended in reviews of the cocaine treatment literature,[1,10-13,20] it is multimodal and adapted to the particular problem areas presented by our patients.

RESULTS

At the time we were preparing this paper, 448 of the proposed subject sample of 450 patient volunteers had been admitted to the program, 423 in time to have completed three months in our randomized, controlled comparison of INT, IND, and IND-GRP treatments. Regarding cocaine use; subject/patients met DSM-III-R Criteria and were judged to exhibit, on average, seven of the nine DSM-III-R Substance Use Dependence Criteria. They reported having used for approximately seven years.

The average ASI drug severity score was 6.3 ± 1.2 and the number of prior drug treatments was 1.0 ± 1.3. The most common second drug was alcohol (45.4%) and only 3.3% reported current IV use of cocaine. Urinalyses at admission were positive for cocaine in 48.1% and other drugs in 8.5%. The proportion of cocaine positive urines was associated negatively with referral from a controlled environment such as hospital, jail, or shelter ($X^2 = 13.57$, df = 4, p < .01) and positively with the number of days used in the last 30 (F = 2.30, df = 4, 340, p < .02).

Testing the randomization procedure for the current sample, comparisons of IND, INT, and IND-GRP on over 90 intake variables revealed three significant differences which is what one would expect on the basis of chance alone.

For our measure of retention we settled on the number of calendar days, inclusive, between the first and last visits to the clinic. It is comparable across treatment modalities which require scheduling different weekly rates of treatment visits. It correlates very highly ($r \geq$ .89) with the proportion of scheduled visits attended and, within modalities, with the number of actual visits attended.

In-Treatment Functioning

Results with regard to the overall effectiveness of treatment were not at all inconsistent with previous research, indicating that persons remaining in treatment longer did better. The treatment plans developed at intake included in order of importance, those problems the patient wished to address during treatment. Treatment plan updates at months 1, 2, and 3 (i.e., end-of-treatment) show the degree of improvement noted for these problems as well as for substance use (general) and cocaine use on 7-point scales (1 = no improvement; 3 = slight; 5 = moderate; 7 = problem resolution). For those research patients who remained in treatment at 1 month, 2 months, and 3 months (i.e., decreasing Ns), average personal problem improvement increased from 3.79 ± 1.55 to 3.96 ± 1.52 to 4.78 ± 1.48, while substance abuse improved (i.e., scores increased) from 4.81 ± 2.07 to 5.31 ± 2.05 to 6.01 ± 1.63, and cocaine use improved from 5.24 ± 2.04 to 6.01 ± 1.59 to 6.32 ± 1.33. Moreover, the proportion of individuals remaining in treatment who gave a positive urine decreased sharply over the 3 months from 22.6% in the first month, to 13.7% in the second month to 5.7% in the third month.

Despite the overall improvement that occurred, however, no differences were found in the above comparisons in relation to treatment modality (IND, IND-GRP, INT).

For the groups combined, improvement at one month on the problems noted by patients to be important to them was associated with longer program retention (r = .24, n = 173, p < .01) and with a greater number of negative urines (r = .26, n = 173, p < .001). The longer individuals remained in treatment the more likely were their last urine samples before leaving to have tested negative. For example, those whose last urine sample before leaving the program was negative for cocaine (N = 163) had stayed an average of 43.9 days while those whose last urine was positive (N = 139) had stayed an average of 20.7 days (t = 6.88, p < .001). As treatment retention increased, the proportion of last urine positives decreased across five periods of retention from 64.2% for 1-3 day dropouts to 9.3% for program completers. This yielded an ordered X^2 = 37.6, 1 df for trend, p > .001.

In sum, individuals showing early improvement on their initially self-identified personal problems such as family relationships, housing, medical/psychiatric, etc., remained in treatment longer. Similarly, for those patients remaining in treatment, mean ratings at 1-month, 2-month, and 3-month treatment plan updates indicated improvement with respect to personal problems and drug use while the proportion of individuals providing dirty urines decreased. Repeated measures analyses would not be appropriate for these comparisons (decreasing Ns), and the results could be interpreted as compatible with either a treatment effect or a consequence of individuals doing well electing to remain in the program while those doing poorly dropped out. There were no differences in our in-treatment results by treatment modality. That is, patients randomly assigned to IND, IND-GRP and INT did equally well.

Treatment Completion

As of this writing, 423 of the proposed sample of 450 patients were admitted in time to have completed the 12-week treatment program. The overall completion rate was 18.2%: 24 of the 144 individuals in IND (16.7%), 23 of the 142 in IND-GRP (16.2%) and 30 of the 137 in INT (21.9%). The difference was not significant. The overall mean time in treatment was 33.40 days with 35.06 for IND, 31.99 for IND-GRP, and 33.14 days for INT and these were not significantly different. If we excluded from analyses those individuals who did not complete intake and at least one equivalent week of treatment (i.e., 1 visit in IND, 2 in IND-GRP, and 3 in INT) the percentage of completers increases from 18.2% to 29.3% and time in treatment increases from 33.4 to 47.8 days.

For the 58 volunteers who at this time had completed both intake and end-of-treatment assessments, significant improvement was found on the ASI Drug, Alcohol, Legal, Family, and Psychological composite measures, and the number of days of cocaine used in the last 30 days. No significant differences were found from intake to completion in medical condition, employment status, and in the numbers of volunteers living in controlled environments (i.e., shelter, recovery houses, etc.) in the previous 30 days. In addition, there were significant differences on the Beck Depression Inventory and on all scales of the SCL-90-R (Table 1).

TABLE 1. Improvement Intake to Treatment Completion, for All Volunteers Completing the 12-Week Program and Pre-and Post-Evaluations.

	All Volunteers				
	Intake		Completion		
	M	SD	M	SD	P
Drug Use and ASI Composites					
Days coc/30	6.0	7.9	.46	1.21	.001
ASI: Medic	.35	.32	.43	.32	ns
ASI: Empl	.85	.22	.82	.23	ns
ASI: Alco	.19	.20	.10	.10	.001
ASI: Drug	.17	.07	.11	.06	.001
ASI: Legal	.14	.19	.07	.15	.005
ASI: Fam/S	.26	.19	.18	.15	.005
ASI: Psych	.27	.22	.18	.20	.05
Controlled Environment/ 30 days	5.4	10.1	7.2	12.8	ns
Psychiatric Symptomatology					
Beck Depress	15.2	9.6	6.3	6.5	.001
SCL: Somat	55.9	11.6	52.2	11.9	.05
SCL: Obs/Comp	61.8	11.9	56.2	11.8	.001
SCL: Int Sens	63.6	12.0	57.2	11.5	.001
SCL: Depress	63.5	11.9	55.2	12.3	.001
SCL: Anxiety	60.7	13.3	53.5	12.7	.001
SCL: Hostil	58.5	11.6	53.1	11.2	.001
SCL: Phob Anx	61.3	11.3	57.4	11.3	.05
SCL: Paranoid	61.6	13.3	55.9	11.7	.001
SCL: Psychot	65.5	12.0	59.0	10.8	.001

However, despite the large number of highly significant differences from beginning to end of treatment, there were no differences found by treatment modality (IND, IND-GRP, INT) on any of our outcome measures recorded at treatment completion (Table 2).

Similarly, among the 58 persons completing both intake and end-of-treatment assessments, we found that an average of 9.4% were referred to be seen by the program psychiatrist at some time during their treatment, 5.7% required pharmacotherapy and 17% received additional individual treatment during the three month treatment period. None of these ancillary service needs differed across treatment modalities (Table 2).

Utilizing the 7-point scale, defined earlier, counselor ratings of cocaine use at the end of treatment indicated that at that time there was little cocaine use reported (average rating 6.25 ± 1.29). While

TABLE 2. Treatment Completion Scores, Compared Across Treatment Modalities.

	All Volunteers		Individual		Ind & Group		Intensive		p*
	M %	SD	M %	SD	M %	SD	M %	SD	
Drug Use and ASI Composites									
Days coc/30	0.46	1.20	0.71	1.61	0.21	0.63	0.48	1.21	ns
ASI: Medic	0.42	0.32	0.35	0.33	0.49	0.28	0.41	0.34	ns
ASI: Empl	0.81	0.23	0.72	0.30	0.84	0.19	0.86	0.19	ns
ASI: Alco	0.10	0.10	0.09	0.11	0.10	0.11	0.11	0.09	ns
ASI: Drug	0.11	0.06	0.11	0.08	0.10	0.05	0.11	0.06	ns
ASI: Legal	0.07	0.15	0.07	0.15	0.04	0.09	0.09	0.18	ns
ASI: Fam/S	0.17	0.15	0.14	0.16	0.17	0.13	0.20	0.16	ns
ASI: Psych	0.18	0.21	0.16	0.19	0.16	0.21	0.22	0.23	ns
Controlled Environment/30 days	6.91	12.6	4.00	10.6	1.72	7.06	13.9	15.1	ns
Psychiatric Symptomatology									
Beck Depress	6.31	6.45	7.07	5.91	4.11	4.28	7.85	8.08	ns
SCL: Somat	52.2	11.9	53.5	12.0	51.1	10.7	52.0	13.1	ns
SCL: Obs/Comp	56.2	11.8	57.1	8.0	56.0	12.2	55.6	14.5	ns
SCL: Int Sens	57.2	11.5	59.7	7.9	53.6	13.0	58.2	12.4	ns
SCL: Depress	55.2	12.3	56.5	7.7	50.3	12.3	58.5	14.4	ns
SCL: Anxiety	53.5	12.7	56.0	11.6	49.3	11.3	55.2	14.2	ns
SCL: Hostil	53.1	11.2	53.7	8.5	51.6	12.1	54.0	12.7	ns
SCL: Phob Anx	57.4	11.3	56.6	8.8	54.2	11.9	60.9	12.1	ns
SCL: Paranoid	55.9	11.7	57.3	7.4	54.8	13.9	55.6	12.8	ns
SCL: Psychot	59.0	10.8	59.7	8.3	58.7	11.3	58.6	12.6	ns

End of Treatment
Counselor Ratings and Extra Tx

Coc use rating	6.25	1.29	5.92	1.93	6.42	0.90	6.35	1.06	ns
Av Pos urine/12	0.15	0.29	0.21	0.35	0.21	0.34	0.07	0.14	ns
Prob aver Imprv	5.22	1.30	4.99	1.56	5.59	0.99	5.13	1.30	ns
Psych eval Mo 3	9.4%		6.3%		7.1%		13.0%		ns
Pharmacoth Mo 3	5.7%		0.0%		7.1%		8.1%		ns
Addl Ind Tx Mo 3	17.0%		12.5%		17.1%		26.1%		ns

N of all above   58

those persons receiving INT treatment gave the fewest positive weekly urines (12 possible), 0.07 ± 0.14 compared to 0.21 ± 0.35 (IND) and 0.21 ± 0.34 (IND-GRP), the difference was not significant by modality.

We also found marked improvement in counselor ratings for the average of the three personal problems identified by the patients as important to them when developing their initial treatment plans $(5.22 \pm 1.30$, 7-point scale). Again, with respect to cocaine use (reported and assessed), and problem improvement there were no significant differences across the treatment modalities (Table 2).

Finally it should be noted that all of the patients who completed the program and pre-and post-testing were given favorable discharge ratings (positive prognoses) by their counselors. There were again, no differences by modality.

DISCUSSION

The number of intensive outpatient treatment programs has grown markedly since we instituted our program in 1988. Initially championed by Washton,[14,21] the modality in various modifications has been adopted by many cocaine treatment providers and espoused as an important modality for treating cocaine dependence.[22-24] It is now included among the levels of care described in the ASAM[25] and Cleveland[26] placement criteria. Although it's popularity continues to increase and clinicians seem to believe that intensive outpatient treatment is providing necessary and valuable addiction treatment, to our knowledge, there are no previous reported controlled studies comparing it's effectiveness with traditional, individual counseling.

Consistent with our expectations we found that those persons remaining in treatment longest were more likely to have improved most in their self-identified problem areas and were less likely to have given a last cocaine positive urine. However, none of these improvements, differentiated among the treatment modalities.

We found that for those patients who completed the program, there was significant improvement from intake to end-of-treatment assessments on the ASI, Beck, and the SCL-90. There were no differences, however, according to treatment modality (IND, IND-

GRP, INT). It should be noted that since we did not randomly assign subjects to different lengths of time in treatment, retention could be an effect of treatment, or of "better motivated" patients staying longer, or some combination.

While the overall completion rate across all modalities was not particularly impressive, if the analyses were restricted to those persons completing at least a one-week equivalent of treatment, completion rates improved markedly.

In discussions among the members of our research team there was general agreement that the results were valuable in demonstrating the significance of behavioral change, in essence, the impact of a treatment experience which can really only occur when a patient remains long enough for treatment to have an effect. Staff members were rather surprised that Intensive Treatment did not demonstrate better outcome results than the other modalities of care (as most believed would be the case).

Even after being informed about our data, staff found it very difficult to believe that Intensive Treatment was not better for our patients than the other two modalities. We began to look at and compare the available data for the Individual and Intensive treatments in an effort to locate a source for their belief. One finding was that there were more drop outs very early in Intensive Treatment (Figure 1). Thereafter we found that more of those people who did not drop out early from Intensive Treatment tended to remain in the groups and to complete the program of care as compared to those assigned to Individual who dropped out regularly throughout the 12 week course of the program leaving well defined gaps in counselor's schedules. The "curves" cross at about 6 weeks and at 12 weeks there were more completers in Intensive than Individual but the difference was not significant. Also, because the Intensive groups were not closed, patients were added steadily, leaving the staff with a superficial impression that there was more patient involvement or better retention in the Intensive modality.

As related to our staff's perception of differential treatment effectiveness the information described above seems to indicate that: Firstly, patients dropping out of relatively full, regularly replenished, active INT groups were not as noticeable as were patients who left a one-hour gap in a counselor's appointment schedule

FIGURE 1. Treatment Retention by Time Intervals

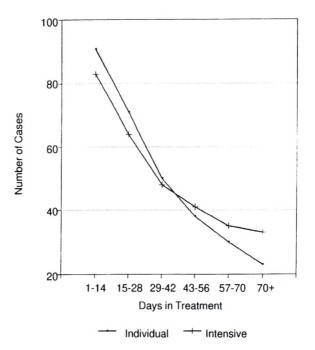

(IND); and, secondly, more patients, although not significantly more, actually did complete Intensive rather than Individual treatment. Also, completion of Intensive is recognized and celebrated by the group members as a marker event while Individual treatment completion is recognized only by counselor and patient. Taken collectively these points may explain why the staff consistently perceived greater effectiveness of Intensive treatment.

Future analyses and reports will include nine-month after intake follow-up comparisons on a wide variety of outcome variables for patients treated in each of the three modalities, an analysis of changes in HIV knowledge and test status from intake to follow-up, and a comparison of improvement in drug use with improvement in AIDS risky behaviors.

Finally, since this project was not designed to match appropriate patients with the most correct treatment modality, a logical next "step" in the research would be to systematically compare those persons who do best in each of the modalities in order to find a set of variables which can effectively help us to match a patient to a treatment in which he/she is most likely to remain. If retention can be maximized the effectiveness of a treatment exposure can be magnified, since to put it succinctly, those who stay in treatment get the most out of treatment.

REFERENCES

1. Siegel RK. Cocaine smoking. Journal on Psychoactive Drugs 1982; 14: 277-359.

2. Siegel RK. Cocaine smoking disorders: Diagnosis and treatment. Psychiatric Annals 1984; 14: 728-732.

3. Weinstein SP, Gottheil E, Smith RH, Migrala KA. Cocaine users seen in medical practice. American Journal of Drug and Alcohol Abuse 1986; 12: 341-354.

4. Extein IL. An update on cocaine. Currents in Affective Illness 1988; 7: 5-13.

5. Weinberg DS, Murray HW. Coping with AIDS: The special problems of New York City. New England Journal of Medicine 1987; 317(23), 1469-1473.

6. Howell DL (ed.). Addicts alter patterns of drug use easier than they do sexual habits. Drugs and Drug Abuse Education Newsletter 1988; 19: 71-76.

7. Fineberg HV. The social dimensions of AIDS. Scientific American 1988; 259: 128-134.

8. Bencivengo MR. Comprehensive Plan for Drug and Alcohol Abuse Treatment and Prevention: Fiscal Year 1988-89 Update. Philadelphia: Department of Public Health, 1989, pp. 1-53.

9. Kleber HD. Cocaine abuse: Historical, epidemiological and psychological perspectives. Journal of Clinical Psychiatry 1988; 49: 3-6.

10. Kleber HD, Gawin FH. Cocaine abuse: A review of current and experimental treatments. NIDA Research Monograph Series, 50. Washington DC: US Government Printing Office, 1984; 111-129.

11. Millman RB. Evaluation and clinical management of cocaine abusers. Journal of Clinical Psychiatry 1988; 49: 27-33.

12. O'Brien CP, Childress AR, Arndt IO, McLellan AT, Woody GE, Moony I. Pharmacological and behavioral treatments of cocaine dependence: Controlled studies. Journal of Clinical Psychiatry 1988; 49: 17-22.

13. Washton AM. Nonpharmacologic treatment of cocaine abuse. Psychiatric Clinics of North America 1986; 9: 563-571.

14. Washton AM. Outpatient treatment techniques. In: Washton AM, Gold MJ. eds. Cocaine: A Clinician's Handbook. New York: Guilford Press, 1987.

15. Milcom Systems. Milcom. Libertyville, IL: Milcom Systems, Hollister Inc., 1989.

16. McLellan AT, Luborsky L, O'Brien CP. Improved diagnostic instrument for substance abuse patients: The Addiction Severity Index. Journal of Nervous and Mental Diseases 1980; 168:26-33.

17. McLellan AT, Luborsky L, Cacciola J, Griffith J, Evans F. New data from the Addiction Severity Index: Reliability and validity in three centers. Journal of Nervous and Mental Diseases 1985; 173:412-423.

18. Beck AT. Cognitive Therapy and the Emotional Disorders. New York, NY: International Universities Press, 1976.

19. DeRogatis L, Lepman R, Rickels K. The Hughes Symptom Check List (HSCL): A self-report symptom inventory. Behavioral Science 1974; 19: 1-16.

20. McLellan AT, Alterman AI, Cacciola J, Metzger D, O'Brien CP. A new measure of substance abuse treatment: Initial studies of the treatment services review. Journal of Nervous and Mental Diseases 1992; 180:101-110.

21. Washton AM. Cocaine Addiction: Treatment, Recovery and Relapse Prevention. New York, NY: W.W. Norton and Co., 1989.

22. Kang SY, Kleinman PH, Woody GE, Millman RB, Todd TC, Kemp J, Lipton DS. Outcomes for cocaine abusers after once-a-week psychosocial therapy. American Journal of Psychiatry 1991; 148:630-635.

23. McAuliffe WE, Albert J. Clean start: An Outpatient Program for Initiating Cocaine Recovery. New York, NY: The Guilford Press, 1992.

24. Rawson RA. The Neurobehavioral Treatment Model: An Outpatient Model for Cocaine Addiction Treatment. Beverly Hills, CA: Matrix Center, 1989.

25. American Society of Addiction Medicine. Patient Placement Criteria for the Treatment of Psychoactive Substance Use Disorders. Washington, D.C. ASAM, 1991.

26. Hoffman NG, Halikas JA, Mee-Lee D. The Cleveland Admission, Discharge, and Transfer Criteria: Model for Chemical Dependency Treatment Programs. Cleveland, Ohio: The Greater Cleveland Hospital Association, 1987.

"Intensive" Outpatient Substance Abuse Treatment: Comparisons with "Traditional" Outpatient Treatment

A. Thomas McLellan, PhD
Teresa Ann Hagan, PhD
Kathleen Meyers, MS
Mary Randall, MS
Jack Durell, MD

SUMMARY. Do "intensive," freestanding outpatient substance abuse treatment programs actually provide more intensive services than "traditional" outpatient programs? Three hundred and thirty-eight patients in 6 "intensive" outpatient (IO) programs (three or more times weekly) were compared with 580 patients from 10 "traditional" outpatient (TO) programs (one or two times weekly) on severity of admission problems, treatment services received and six month outcomes. Results:

A. Thomas McLellan, Teresa Ann Hagan, Kathleen Meyers, Mary Randall and Jack Durell are affiliated with the Treatment Research Institute and the Penn-VA Center for Studies of Addiction, Philadelphia, PA.

Address correspondence to: A. Thomas McLellan, PhD, Treatment Research Institute, 2005 Market Street, One Commerce Square, Suite 1120, Philadelphia, PA 19103.

Prepared as part of an ASAM sponsored symposium on Treatment Outcome in Substance Abuse, January-1995. Additional support was received from ongoing NIAAA, NIDA, CSAT and Veterans Administration research grants to the authors.

[Haworth co-indexing entry note]: "'Intensive' Outpatient Substance Abuse Treatment: Comparisons with 'Traditional' Outpatient Treatment." McLellan, A. Thomas et al. Co-published simultaneously in *Journal of Addictive Diseases* (The Haworth Medical Press, an imprint of The Haworth Press, Inc.) Vol. 16, No. 2, 1997, pp. 57-84; and: *Intensive Outpatient Treatment for the Addictions* (ed: Edward Gottheil, and Barry Stimmel) The Haworth Medical Press, an imprint of The Haworth Press, Inc., 1997, pp. 57-84. Single or multiple copies of this article are available for a fee from The Haworth Document Delivery Service [1-800-342-9678, 9:00 a.m. - 5:00 p.m. (EST). E-mail address: getinfo@haworth.com].

1. IO subjects generally had the most severe medical, employment, legal and psychiatric problems at admission.
2. IO patients received more alcohol and drug focused services; but *fewer* medical and employment focused services than the TO patients. Both groups received very few psychosocial services.
3. There were not significant differences between the IO and TO program samples at follow-up. However, both groups showed significant reductions in substance use, improvements in personal health and social function. *[Article copies available for a fee from The Haworth Document Delivery Service: 1-800-342-9678. E-mail address: getinfo@haworth.com]*

INTRODUCTION

The past few years have witnessed major debate regarding how to stem the increasing costs of health care in this country; particularly the escalating costs of treatments for alcohol and drug dependence. In our view, two forces have been quite influential in recent national efforts to curtail these costs. The first force is the growth of "managed care" companies. Managed care has become the general term for the wide variety of treatment provider and treatment manager entities that seek to reduce costs to the payers (insurance company, self-insured company or state authority) by negotiating a fixed, "per capita" cost to provide all health services–or often just "carved out" mental health and addiction services–to a target patient population. This "per capita" charge is estimated from the likely utilization rates of the population, and the projected costs for the types of services that will be available to the population under the managed care contract. In turn, managed care firms can control the costs of care that they purchase by retaining decision authority regarding *whether* a patient needs a particular type of care (e.g., "pre-certification" of inpatient hospitalization) and *when* there has been adequate amounts of care delivered (e.g., "continuing review" authorizations). It is clear that these, now common practices have dramatically changed the manner in which substance abuse and mental health treatments are now delivered in this country and it is equally clear that these managed care practices have resulted in significant savings for payers.[1,2]

Perhaps surprisingly, a second force that has been influential in reducing the costs of substance abuse treatment is the body of research comparing the effectiveness and costs of inpatient and outpatient forms of that treatment. It has always been accepted that inpatient care, particularly within hospital settings is the most expensive of the various types of substance abuse treatments.[3] However, it was also assumed that this more intensive form of care was also the most effective, particularly with those most severely affected alcohol and drug dependent patients. However, over the past decade, there have been a number of comparative studies that have failed to show significant differences in outcome between inpatient and various forms of outpatient treatment.[4-7] While it is possible to criticize all of these studies on methodolgic, clinical and practical grounds,[8] in fact the *absence* of research findings indicating better outcomes from inpatient than various forms of outpatient substance abuse treatment has provided a *positive* "justification" for the now common practices of the managed care companies to "divert" patients seeking inpatient treatment into a relatively new form of substance abuse treatment, "intensive outpatient" care.

Because of the importance of these cost cutting efforts to the substance abuse treatment field, because of the rapid growth of "intensive" outpatient care, and because of the lack of evaluation studies in this area, we have undertaken the present examination of "intensive" outpatient substance abuse treatment. The paper is presented in two parts. In the first part of this effort, we have attempted to define intensive outpatient care functionally against the reference modalities of day-hospital and "traditional" outpatient care. Here we considered parameters of treatment such as the setting in which the program resides, the planned length of treatment, the frequency of treatment sessions per week, the duration of these sessions each week and the number and types of treatment services provided within these sessions.

In the second part of the paper we used these operational definitions to select representative examples of "intensive outpatient" (IO) and "traditional outpatient" (TO) treatment programs from our national database of treatment programs that have received our standard outcome evaluation.[9] In each of these groups, data were available describing the nature and severity of patients' admission problems, the number and types of services provided to patients during treatment, and their six-month outcomes on a range of substance abuse and social functioning indicators. The paper thus examines "intensive" and "traditional" outpatient treatments as they are delivered in real world programs, in a functional analysis of the similarities and differences between these two forms of substance abuse treatment.

PART I–
DEFINING "INTENSIVE" OUTPATIENT TREATMENT

The American Society of Addiction Medicine (ASAM) has given great thought to the categorization of substance abuse treatments.[10] They have considered at least six parameters in developing their categories of treatment programs. These include the setting of the program (i.e., hospital, residential, etc.), support systems available within the care setting, staff types and qualifications, therapies available within the program, the types of patient assessments used by the program and the level of treatment documentation. Using these parameters, ASAM has defined "intensive outpatient" treatments in their general category called Level II treatments. Notable features of this category include the requirement that the programs in the category have sessions at least three days per week and that the total time spent in treatment each week must equal 9 or more hours. In addition to the freestanding intensive programs, this Level II category also includes "day-hospital" and "evening hospital" programs which are acknowledged to differ from the others within the category by virtue of their hospital setting, the availability of more medical and nursing staff, and generally more treatment hours and services. Interestingly, the ASAM category does not differentiate these Level II programs by therapeutic objective, for example, detoxification, rehabilitation, or relapse prevention.

Using the ASAM definition of "intensive" outpatient treatment as a starting point we performed a search of the available research literature on intensive outpatient substance abuse treatments. The majority of programs identified by this review were "traditional" outpatient substance abuse treatment programs that met once or twice weekly for one to two months. The target population of these programs was usually, recently detoxified patients (often patients who had completed short-term inpatient treatments) and the focus of the program was almost exclusively upon the alcohol and drug use problems of the patients rather than their attendant medical, emotional and social problems. The treatment components provided within these programs typically included 12-step based group counseling sessions focused upon the maintenance of sobriety, alcohol and drug education sessions and individual counseling sessions that were similar in content to the group sessions. Many of these programs also included one or more family sessions or outings, again designed to foster support for sobriety in the home. Because of the prevalence of these programs geographically and the fact that they have been a generic form of treatment in the substance abuse field for more than two decades, we refer to them here as "traditional" outpatient programs.

For the sake of comparison, we were also able to find studies of "day-hospital" treatments.[4-7] Day-hospital care in these studies was typically characterized by daily (at least 5 days per week) treatment sessions, lasting typically 4-6 hours, over a planned treatment duration of 30 to 60 days, all occurring within an outpatient clinic of a medical or psychiatric hospital. As described by Alterman et al.,[7] this form of treatment appears to have been designed to provide the same types and amounts of services that are typically available within a hospital setting–without the bed costs. Thus, the treatment sessions described in the Alterman et al. study[7] contained a range of services such as group and individual counseling directed at the alcohol and drug problems of the patients as well as appointments with medical and nursing staff for related medical disorders, therapy sessions by psychologists and/or psychiatrists focused upon the emotional problems of the patients, and additional appointments with social work staff focused upon the living arrangements, employment and/or self-support. In fact Alterman and colleagues have shown in their Veterans Administration study, the cost of these "day-hospital" services were approximately three-fifths of the corresponding inpatient hospital costs.[7]

Operational Definitions–Although the ASAM Level II criteria had included day and evening hospital programs in the same category as other "intensive" outpatient programs our review of the literature and our examination of our own database suggested important differences between those outpatient programs located within hospital settings, and those that were freestanding. For example, most of the freestanding treatment programs that could be categorized as "intensive" by the ASAM criteria, did not have a "working relationship with a medical provider,"[10, p. 26] although consultation was usually available. In contrast, all the day-hospital programs in our literature review and in our database had at least one full time physician on staff and most had at least one full time nurse. Most of the freestanding Level II programs did not have a "direct affiliation with more/less intensive levels of care," nor the "ability to conduct or arrange needed laboratory tests."[10, p. 26] Consequently, the majority of the day-hospital treatment programs in our reviews admitted alcohol and cocaine dependent patients who were still suffering from physiological withdrawal and/or instability. In contrast, the great majority of the freestanding programs had chosen to focus their efforts on the rehabilitation of patients who had been previously detoxified or stabilized at another program. These seemed to be important clinical and administrative differences within the ASAM Level II category of intensive programs and we chose to focus our report on the freestanding examples of intensive outpatient care.

Within the freestanding outpatient programs, we relied upon the ASAM level II criteria to differentiate "intensive" from "traditional" outpatient treatment based upon: the orientation or treatment goals of the program, the planned duration of treatment, the number of sessions per week, the duration of these sessions and the content of these sessions. Thus, we have operationally defined freestanding "intensive outpatient" substance abuse treatment as abstinence oriented care provided *outside a hospital environment*, at a frequency of at least three treatment sessions per week, lasting at least three hours per session, for a planned duration of at least 30 days. Further, consistent with the ASAM guidelines for Level II programs, we have required that these sessions contain more than just services directed only at the substance abuse problems of the patients. We included as "intensive" programs, those that described themselves as offering services for at least two of the following types of problems typically found among substance dependent individuals: medical, family, employment, psychiatric, housing or legal problems. Again, while we have chosen to exclude day-hospital programs from this definition, for the reasons described, all remaining programs in our "intensive" category appear to fit the ASAM Level II category.

We used the same functional parameters to operationally define "traditional" outpatient, abstinence oriented substance abuse treatment programs as those providing care *outside a hospital environment* at a frequency of no more than two treatment sessions per week, lasting no more than two hours per session, for a planned duration of at least 30 days. Consistent with the "traditional" abstinence-focused orientation of these programs, we included as "traditional" programs, those that focused almost entirely upon services directed at the maintenance of sobriety—such as twelve steps, alcohol education, relapse prevention, etc. We have summarized these operational definitions in Table 1.

Representing the Two Types of Programs in the Database—The data base from which the sample programs have been drawn is comprised of information collected on samples of substance abuse patients treated in standard substance abuse programs over the past eight years. Data derive from studies staff at the Center for Studies of Addiction at the University of Pennsylvania and from the standard protocol employed by the Treatment Research Institute.[9] The database is one of the largest and most comprehensive collections of pre-, during- and post-treatment data presently available. In all cases, only data from trained interviewers have been used and all of these data have been screened to eliminate inaccurate or improperly collected information. Finally, only data collected from independent evaluators rather than program personnel have been used to develop the outcome evaluation, thus eliminating clinical bias in the determination of efficacy.

All data were collected following an "intent to treat" paradigm evaluating randomly or consecutively selected samples of 50-100 patients who were admitted to a treatment program and following all of these patients, regardless of whether or when they exited treatment. This design provides an estimate of the outcomes of care for the "average" patient who enters the program—rather than a description of outcomes solely among those who have complied fully with care (i.e., "completers"). The procedures used to follow patients in these protocols are described below.

TABLE 1. Functional Contrast of "Intensive" and "Traditional" Outpatient Substance Abuse Treatment Programs

Program Parameter	Intensive Outpatient	Shared Components	Traditional Outpatient
Setting		Non-Hospital	
Orientation		Total Abstinence	
Duration	30-90 Days		45-60 Days
Sessions Per Week	3-5 per week		1-2 per week
Hours Per Session	4-6 hours		1-2 hours
Content of Sessions		Group/Ind Sobriety Counseling	
		12-Steps	
		Relapse Prevention	
		Alcohol Education	
	2-5 Medical Appts.		0-1 Medical Appts.
	2-6 Family Therapy		0-2 Family Therapy
	3-9 Psychotherapy		0-2 Psychotherapy
	2-4 Emp. Counseling		0 Emp. Counseling
	0-4 Housing/Support Sessions		0 Housing/Support Sessions

64

In the present study we have focused upon treatment programs that were designed to provide rehabilitation oriented treatment toward a goal of abstinence from both alcohol and drugs. For these reasons we did not include methadone maintenance programs or programs that provided only detoxification. Four of the remaining programs were hospital based and were thus considered "day-hospital" programs. Eleven other outpatient programs were not included because they had treatment durations that were too short (e.g., 15-30 days), or because they were developed for specific, non-representative populations (e.g., probationers, parolees, pregnant women, adolescents, psychiatrically ill substance abusers). Five programs were excluded because their characteristics did not clearly suggest one of the two categories of interest.

Thus, sixteen outpatient, abstinence-oriented treatment programs meeting the above inclusion/exclusion criteria were included in the analyses. Ten of these were "traditional" programs, seven private and three public; and six were "intensive" programs, three public and three private. None of the private programs received any state or federal funding for administration or operation, while at least half of the public programs received federal, state or city funding to defray some of the services provided (e.g., AIDS prevention counseling, counseling for pregnant women, etc.) *It is important to note* that all 16 programs were from the northeast section of the country thus it is not possible to infer that the data would be representative of the national treatment system.

PART II–
COMPARISON OF INTENSIVE
AND OUTPATIENT TREATMENT PROGRAMS
DATA COLLECTION METHODS

The same core battery of evaluation instruments and research procedures was used in each of the treatment programs and for all subjects. Participation for all subjects was voluntary. Subjects were told that they would be interviewed in person at the start of treatment, by telephone either weekly or bi-weekly during their treatment, and again, seven months following treatment admission (regardless of whether they completed treatment). Acceptance rates ranged from 65% to 90%.

Patient Measures at Admission to Treatment–Patients were interviewed at treatment admission using the Addiction Severity Index (ASI).[11-13] The ASI is a 45-60 minute structured interview that measures the lifetime and recent (past 30 days) severity of problems in seven areas commonly affected among alcohol and drug dependent individuals. These include medical status, employment, alcohol use, drug use, crime, family/social relationships and psychiatric symptoms.

In each of these areas, items measuring the severity of the problem during the previous 30 days are combined into a composite or factor score that gives a general measure of problem severity.[12,13] These composites are computer scored with values ranging from 0 (no significant problem) to 1.0 (extreme problem). The ASI has been repeatedly found to offer reliable and valid measures of patient status in each of the problem areas in opiate, alcohol and cocaine abusing populations.[13]

Treatment Content Measures–While the ASI measures the nature and severity of treatment problems presented by the patient at the start of treatment and later at follow-up, the nature and number of treatment services actually received by patients for those problems during the course of their rehabilitation was measured by the Treatment Services Review (TSR).[14] The TSR is also a technician administered interview that requires 5-10 minutes to complete and is administered to each patient weekly or bi-weekly, usually over the phone during the course of treatment. The TSR provides a simple and reliable quantitative record of the number of professional services (specialized therapy or treatment sessions, medications, etc.) and discussion sessions (group or individual counseling) that each patient received in each of the same seven problem areas covered by the ASI.[14] For example, in the medical section, subjects were asked to report the number of times in the prior week they had seen a doctor, a nurse, received a prescription for a medication, received any type of medical testing, or had a significant discussion related to their medical problems with a counselor or other member of the program staff. The TSR measures both the services that are provided within the program and through referral at other programs or agencies.

Outcome Measurement–Patients were contacted seven months from their admission to treatment and since the great majority of subjects in these programs had completed their treatment within 30 days, we refer to the follow-up as a six-month post treatment follow-up. Follow-up efforts were begun two weeks prior to the exact anniversary data and were extended two weeks following that point in the event that a patient was not able to be located. The follow-up ASI required approximately 20 minutes and was again administered by a trained residential technician who was not part of the treatment process. Subjects were paid $15 for their time required to complete the follow-up interview. Approximately 79% of patients across all programs were successfully interviewed during the "follow-up" window using these techniques and that ranged from a high of 98% to a low of 67%. Follow-up contact rates were not different between the IO and TO samples.

There were several methods for insuring information validity built into the follow-up interview. First, subjects were repeatedly assured that their information would not be communicated to any individual or agency. Second, subjects were told that they did not have to answer a question with which they were uncomfortable, or provide information that they wished to keep private. These two aspects of the interview procedure provided confidentiality reassurance as well as an additional answer option for the subject in lieu of falsification. Third, there are a number of information cross-checks in the interview and technicians were trained to notice and respond to inconsistencies. Sections of the ASI that the interviewer felt were compromised by failure to understand or by purposeful distortion were not used in the data analyses. Where three or more sections were compromised the entire interview was eliminated. We discarded 27 follow-up interviews due to three or more invalid sections and these were spread approximately evenly across all the programs and populations represented.

Outcome Domains–As we have suggested elsewhere,[15,16] we typically consider four outcome domains that we feel are relevant both to the rehabilitative goals of the patient and to the public health and safety goals of society:

1. *Reduction of Alcohol and Drug Use.* This is the foremost goal of all substance abuse treatments.
2. *Improved Personal Health.* Improvements in the medical and psychiatric health of substance abusing patients are clearly important from a healthcare utilization perspective but in addition, improvements in these areas are also related to prevention of relapse to substance abuse.
3. *Improved Social Function.* Improvements in the social function of substance abusing patients are important from a societal benefit perspective but they too, are related to prevention of relapse.
4. *Reduction in Public Safety Threats.* The threats to public safety from substance abusing individuals come from behaviors that spread infectious diseases and from the commission of personal and property crimes. In this study we were not able to measure AIDS and TB risk behaviors and so this domain is only represented by measures of crime.

RESULTS

What Were the Background Characteristics of the Patients in These Two Types of Programs at the Start of Treatment?–Subjects were 918 adults admitted to treatment in the programs described above and successfully contacted at follow-up. They are described in Table 2, by treatment category. As can be seen, the patients admitted to these programs were approximately 41 years old and primarily male and European American, with a high school education and a history of approximately four prior treatments for alcohol and drug dependence. The total sample averaged 7 years of problematic alcohol use (intoxication at least three times per week), four years of regular cocaine use and ten years of regular marijuana use. On average the group had been abstinent a total of only 11 months since beginning regular substance abuse, despite being treated an average of two times for alcohol problems and two times for drug problems.

While the majority of the variables examined indicated that the two groups were more similar than different, there were the expectable indications that the IO patients were somewhat more severely problematic than the TO patients at the time of their treatment

TABLE 2. Patient Background Characteristics at Admission to Treatment

	IO Programs	Sig. Dif.	TO Programs	Total Sample
Number of Patients	338		580	918
DEMOGRAPHIC FACTORS				
Age	40		41	41
% Male	95		97	96
% White	76		78	77
Yrs. Education	12		11	11
# Prior Alcohol Treatments	2		1	2
# Prior Drug Treatments	2		2	2
% Married	45		38	37
% Separated/Divorced	47		43	39
% Living w/Substance Abuser	23	*	11	16
% Unstable Living Arrangements	14		8	11
SUBSTANCE ABUSE				
Yrs. Problematic Alcohol Use	9		6	7
Yrs. Problematic Cocaine Use	5		4	4
Yrs. Problematic Barbituate & Tranquilizer	2		1	1
Yrs. Marijuana Abuse	10		11	11
Longest Pd. of Abstinence (mos.)	9	*	15	12
MEDICAL PROBLEM				
% w/ Chronic Medical Problems	30	**	12	20
Medical Hospitalizations	5		3	4
EMPLOYMENT PROBLEMS				
% w/ Skill or Trade	75		71	73
Longest Pd. of Emp. (yrs.)	5		7	6
% Employed	53	**	68	59
LEGAL PROBLEM				
% Awaiting Charges	11	*	4	8
% Probation/Parole	11		6	8
% Ever Incarcerated	38	**	12	27
PSYCHIATRIC PROBLEM				
% Having Previous Psych. Tmt.	30		23	28
% Attempted Suicide	23	*	13	19
% Reported Lifetime Depression	61	*	42	53
% Reporting Prob. Controlling Violence	34		36	35

* = p < .05, ** = p < .01 (t-test or Chi Square between groups).

admission. Among the first indications of differences between IO and TO patients in these samples is the difference in the proportion of patients who were living in "unstable arrangements" (e.g., homeless) or with someone who was actively abusing drugs or alcohol. In general, while both groups of patients showed substantial histories of alcohol and drug use, the IO patients had somewhat (though not statistically) longer histories of use and a shorter period of abstinence. A statistically and clinically significant difference between the two groups was evident in the medical status at admission with 35% of the IO patients reporting chronic medical problems that continued to interfere with their lives—as compared with only 12% in the TO group. While a majority of both groups had been employed for significant periods, significantly more TO than IO patients had been employed in the month prior to their admission to treatment. More IO than TO patients reported and were currently experiencing legal problems at the time of their admission to treatment. Finally, the IO patients reported more serious and more varied lifetime psychiatric symptoms than those of the TO patients, particularly in the areas of suicidality and depression.

What Services Did These Substance Abuse Treatment Programs Provide?—As described, TSR information was collected from all patients regarding the nature and number of treatment services they received from their program directly, or through referral. In Table 3, we have collapsed both on-site and referred services into a single category for each program. While we actually recorded the frequency of services provided each week, in fact for most categories of services surveyed and for most weeks of those surveys, *most patients reported receiving no services.* Thus, Table 3 reports the average *percentage of patients receiving at least one session or appointment,* in each of the service areas during each week of treatment.

As expected, the majority of patients (in both IO and TO programs) were provided various types of drug and alcohol sessions and services. These sessions, whether group or individual, and whether educational or psychotherapeutic, were all focused upon the goals of motivating and teaching patients to become and remain abstinent. Specifically, group counseling for abstinence and for relapse prevention as well as educational classes were the major treat-

TABLE 3. Proportion of Patients Receiving at Least One Session or Service in Each Category During Treatment

Proportion of Patients Who Received These Services in . . .	IO Programs		TO Programs
ALCOHOL & DRUG SERVICES	%		%
Received Alc/Drug Meds	11		13
Had a Breathalyzer screen	55	*	48
Had a Urine Screen	38		35
Had Alcohol/Drug Education Session	72	*	66
Attended AA/NA–Out of Prog.	65	*	50
Had a Relapse Prev. Session	80	*	68
Had an grp. discussion re: Alc/Drug Probs	94		92
Had an ind. discussion re: Alc/Drug Probs	36		41
MEDICAL SERVICES			
Received Med. Prescription	6	*	11
Was admitted to a hospital	3		1
Saw a Physician	3		1
Saw a Nurse/NP	4		7
EMPLOYMENT SERVICES			
Had an ind. discussion re: Emp Probs	7		9
Saw an Employment Specialist	2	*	11
LEGAL SERVICES			
Had Justice System contacted	2		4
Had an ind. discussion re: Leg Probs	2		6
FAMILY SERVICES			
Had an ind. discussion re: Fam probs	3	*	7
Saw a Family Specialist	1		3
PSYCHIATRIC SERVICES			
Received Psych Meds Prescription	8		3
Had relaxation training	11	*	4
Had Psych testing	2		1
Saw a Psych Specialist	8		6
Had an ind. discussion re: Psy Probs	16		13

* = p < .05 by Z test for differences between proportions.

ment services provided in both types of programs. As can be seen, and as was expected, the IO programs provided breathalyzer screenings for alcohol use, educational sessions, AA sessions and relapse prevention sessions to a significantly greater proportion of patients than the TO programs.

While the frequency of these services is not shown, the IO programs usually offered four to six of these sessions while the TO programs usually offered two or three in the course of a typical week. Individual discussions with counselors regarding specific problems of remaining abstinent were also available in both types of programs but were less frequent and paradoxically, more likely to occur in the TO than in the IO programs–among those patients who received at least one session. The average frequency of individual drug counseling appointments was slightly less than two sessions per week in the IO programs and less than one session per week in the TO programs. Very few patients received anti-craving medications or biological monitoring of recent substance use by breathalyzer or urine test. In fact the average frequency of urine and breath testing was once per month in both types of programs.

Inspection of the remainder of Table 3 shows that very few patients in either of the two program categories received services directed at the additional problems of education, employment, medical or psychological health or family relations in either type of program. Less than 20% of patients in either program category received any professional service or even a counseling session directed toward any of these problems during their treatment. More interesting, is the fact that there were only four statistically significant differences between the proportions of patients receiving services in the "intensive" and "traditional" programs. In fact, in three of the four instances where there were statistically significant differences between the two groups, *the TO programs provided those services to a higher proportion of patients than the IO programs* (this is designated by shading within the boxes around the asterisks). Specifically, the IO patients were more likely than the TO patients to receive psychiatric services, and this was statistically significant in the case of relaxation training. In contrast, the TO patients were significantly more likely to receive a medication prescription from a physician, to see an employment specialist (typically a social worker) and to have an individual discussion or session dedicated to family problems, than those admitted to the IO programs in this sample.

What Were the Outcomes from Substance Abuse Treatment?—Table 4 compares the progress made by patients in both the IO and TO groups as measured by the ASI at intake and at six month follow-up. As previously indicated, we performed an "intent to treat" analysis including all subjects that were accepted for treatment by the programs (i.e., they intended to treat them) regardless of whether they completed treatment. As such, this analysis offers a more conservative evaluation of treatment effects than an evaluation that would be restricted to just those who completed the full course of treatment. Shown in the table are both the ASI composite scores and selected individual items from each of the ASI problem areas. Composite scores range from 0 (no problem) to 1 (extreme problem) and represent the severity of the problems during the 30 days prior to each interview. The ASI measures have been grouped into the four outcome domains previously discussed.

Prior to analyses of the individual outcome measures we performed a between-groups, repeated measures multiple analysis of covariance (MANCOVA) in each outcome domain using the six-month ASI composite scores within each of the domains as the independent variables and the baseline composite scores as the covariates. We performed these general analyses as a conservative test of any overall trends in outcome between the groups and to provide rationale for testing the significance of individual items within each outcome domain. Results of the substance use and personal health MANCOVAs both indicated significant ($p < .01$) improvements from baseline to follow-up across groups, but no between-group differences in the adjusted follow-up scores ($p > .10$). The MANCOVA in the public safety domain showed a marginal within-groups improvement ($p < .08$) and no significant between-groups difference at six months ($p > .10$). Results of the social function MANCOVA indicated significant within-group improvements across groups ($p < .001$) as well as a between-groups difference ($p < .03$) in the adjusted six month follow-up.

We interpreted these results as providing permission to examine the within group changes for all groups on all four domains using

TABLE 4. Pre- to Post-Treatment Changes in Substance Abuse Patients Treated in Intensive and Traditional Outpatient Programs

PROBLEM MEASURE	IO PROGRAMS			TO PROGRAMS			ANCOVA @ 6-MO
	BASELINE N = 338	t	6 MONTHS N = 338	BASELINE N = 580	t	6 MONTHS N = 580	
OUTCOME DOMAIN #1—REDUCTION IN ALCOHOL AND DRUG USE							
Drug Composite Score	.166	***	.065	.148	***	.059	NS
Days Stimulant use	5	**	2	4	**	2	NS
Days Depressant use	2		1	1		1	NS
Alcohol Composite Score	.422	***	.111	.398	***	.096	NS
Days Alcohol use	11	***	4	9	**	3	NS
Days drank to intoxication	9	***	3	7	**	2	NS
OUTCOME DOMAIN #2—INCREASED PERSONAL HEALTH							
Medical Composite Score	.254	**	.197	.189		.191	NS
Days Medical Problems	6		4	4		5	NS
Psychiatric Comp Score	.341	**	.166	.262	**	.121	NS
Days psych problems	9	**	4	7	**	3	NS
OUTCOME DOMAIN #3—IMPROVED SOCIAL FUNCTION							
Employment Comp Score	.755	*	.703	.541	**	.401	**
Days worked in past 30	8		9	13		15	**
Employment Income	$610		$671	$745		$811	*
Family Composite Score	.278	**	.114	.254	*	.211	*
Days family conflicts	5	*	2	3		2	NS
OUTCOME DOMAIN #4—REDUCTION IN PUBLIC SAFETY CONCERNS							
Legal Composite Score	.089		.037	.071		.031	NS
Days illegal activity	3	*	1	1		1	NS
Illegal income	$46		$22	$37		$14	NS

* = p < .05, ** = p < .01 *** = p < .001 (Paired t-tests used within groups—ANCOVA between groups; baseline value was covariate).
All variables reflect the 30 days prior to baseline and 24-week evaluations.
Factor scores vary from 0 to 1; larger values equal greater severity.

74

paired t-tests. The results of these paired t-tests are shown by the asterisks between the baseline and follow-up columns for each of the groups. The results of the MANCOVAs also indicated a rationale for testing between-groups differences *but only within those variables in the social function domain.* The results of the individual ANCOVAs within the social function domain (in each case the baseline value was the covariate) are shown in the last column of Table 4.

As can be seen there is ample evidence that both groups made significant progress following treatment at approximately the same level and in most of the same ASI problem areas. The IO subjects showed significant ($p = .05$ or less) improvements on 12 out of the 18 comparisons, as compared with 9 statistically significant improvements on the 18 criterion variables in the TO group. Both the IO and the TO program groups showed significant reductions in the severity of their drug problem composite scores, due primarily to reductions in the frequency of stimulant (cocaine) use. In addition, both groups showed reductions in alcohol composite scores, in the frequency of *any* alcohol use and in the frequency of alcohol to the point of intoxication (three drinks or more per sitting). While the IO patients entered treatment with somewhat more severe problems and more frequent usage of these substances than the TO patients, both groups made significant improvements and there were no differences between the two groups of patients by the six-month follow-up.

With regard to the outcome domain of personal health, again both groups showed some significant improvements, especially in the psychiatric area. The IO patients showed significant additional improvements in their medical status. ANCOVAs were not performed in this domain since the MANCOVA had not indicated a basis to examine the individual items. In the social function domain, both groups showed significant improvements in the employment composite score. The TO patients exhibited significant improvement in their employment earnings, while the IO patients showed significant improvements in the family composite score and in the days of reported family problems. As shown by the ANCOVAs in this area, there were four significant overall differences between the two groups at six months, and *three of them favored the TO group.*

Specifically, the ANCOVAs on individual items within this domain showed that the TO group had significantly ($p < .05$ or less) better adjusted outcomes in the employment composite score, as well as in the days worked and earned income variables. The IO group had significantly better six month outcome on the Family composite score.

The data from the analysis of the public safety domain indicated that while there was indication of positive change in both groups from admission to follow-up, only the variable of crime days per month showed statistically significant improvement, and only in the IO group. No individual variables were examined for between group differences due to the results of the MANCOVA in this domain.

DISCUSSION

The present paper was initiated as a means of exploring the now pervasive category of freestanding, intensive outpatient substance abuse treatment programs. To this end, we examined samples of these programs from our national database and contrasted these programs against a second sample of "traditional" outpatient programs from the same database on measures of patient status at the start of treatment, the nature and amount of treatment services provided to patients in each problem area, and finally, in terms of the improvements shown by patients in these two types of programs at six-month follow-up.

We began our evaluation of these programs using the ASAM definition of Level II "intensive" outpatient programs.[10] However, we excluded "day-hospital" programs from this definition since we felt that there were sufficient structural and functional differences to keep them separate. Thus, while the programs that have been included here do appear to meet the criteria for ASAM Level II (see Table 1 for a summary), it should be recognized that the potentially more intensive day and evening hospital programs have not been included in these analyses. Using this definition and examples from our database[9] we compared patient samples from six programs designated by us as "intensive" (IO) and ten programs designated by us as "traditional" (TO) outpatient, abstinence oriented treatment for alcohol and/or cocaine dependent individuals (we also eliminated methadone maintenance programs from these analyses). Three findings resulted from this restricted, retrospective evaluation of programs in our database (see Limitations, below).

Patients admitted to IO programs had generally more, and more severe substance use and related social and health problems than patients admitted to TO programs. Consistent with what might have been expected, both groups of substance dependent patients reported significant and multiple substance abuse and substance abuse-related problems at the time of their admission to the index treatment. In general, the IO patients were somewhat more severely affected than the TO patients, particularly in the medical, legal and psychiatric problem areas.

"Intensive" outpatient treatments provide more drug and alcohol counseling sessions than "traditional" outpatient programs; but not more medical, employment, family or social services. In fact, there were indications that IO patients were somewhat less likely to receive medical, employment and family services than TO patients. From our examination of the service profiles of these programs, the drug and alcohol focused services that are the hallmark of most contemporary treatment programs (group therapy, individual counseling for drug and alcohol use, AA/NA, relapse prevention, etc.) were provided at generally greater frequency and to significantly more patients in the IO than in the TO programs. However, IO programs provided very few services for the employment, crime, health, psychological or family problems that were so apparent in these patients (particularly the IO patients) and that were so often the impetus for treatment referral.

Both IO and TO patients showed significant improvements at six month follow-up in the areas of substance use, personal health and social function. In general, there were few differences between the two modalities in outcome at follow-up. Improvements were seen in both the IO and TO treatment samples at about the same magnitude and frequency. Comparisons of the months prior to admission and six-month follow-up in these patients revealed a 60% reduction in days of alcohol use and more than a 50% reduction in days of cocaine use. The outcome results also indicated smaller but important improvements in medical and psychiatric health and in criminal behaviors that were directly linked to substance use. While both groups of patients also showed increased social function as evidenced by increased attendance at work, increased earnings and fewer family and social conflicts, the TO patients had significantly better outcomes in this domain than the IO patients. These data offer an indication that both these forms of substance abuse treatment are "effective" and it is important to note that these findings are not new or unusual in this regard.[3,17-19]

Limitations of the Present Research

As indicated repeatedly in the description of the study, there are some significant limitations to this work that require caution in the interpretation of the findings. Perhaps most importantly, the definitions of "intensive" and "traditional" outpatient programs used in the present examination were admittedly somewhat arbitrary. We did not include "day-hospital" programs in our definition of "intensive" outpatient treatments. It could be argued that we should have included the day-hospital programs in this definition and that by excluding them we have under-represented the effectiveness of generically more intensive outpatient treatment. In fact, this is a good argument. Inspection of the data from the four day-hospital programs we have in our database suggests that the patients who were admitted to these were even more severely and pervasively affected than those in the present IO group, that a greater range and number of services were typically provided to these patients, and that their outcomes are as good or better than those seen in the present IO group. We excluded these programs purposely since they are so different in structure, location, patient mix characteristics and staffing pattern from the free standing intensive outpatient programs that were examined here; and because we had so few representative examples. As our database grows, we hope to perform future studies that will contrast inpatient, day and evening hospital, freestanding intensive outpatient and traditional outpatient programs using the same methods presented here.

An equally important limitation of the present findings is the nature of the database used to evaluate the issue. The great majority of the programs selected came from the northeastern section of the country, representing only eight states. These programs were *not* randomly selected from a master file of all programs in the country but rather, were self-identified by having participated in one of the standard outcome evaluations, conducted either by the Center for Studies of Addiction or as part of a standard outcome evaluation by the Treatment Research Institute. This is very important and it should be very clear that *we cannot generalize these findings to the national level.* Again, it will be important for future studies with more representative samples to examine this issue on a larger scale.

Given these important caveats, it is reasonable to question whether and in what way the data can contribute to our understanding of substance abuse treatment. In this regard, there were a number of positive aspects to the study that give us confidence in the results. For example, all programs were standard programs operating under "real world" conditions and thus offer some indication of the types of patients entering these treatment modalities, the nature and patterns of services provided and the types of outcomes observed at a six-month follow-up. Secondly, all treatment service and follow-up data were collected by research technicians who were independent from the treatment programs and who used instruments and procedures that have been repeatedly tested for reliability and validity in these populations. Follow-up data were collected on 79% of the patients sampled using an intent to treat design, thereby providing a reasonable and somewhat conservative representation of the treatment effects.

A major consideration in all studies employing self-report data is the reliability and validity of the information collected. Several points are relevant here. First, the data collected were based on confidential interviews at admission and follow-up using instruments and procedures that have been validated in many similar studies.[13] Within the primary instrument used (ASI) there are built in consistency checks to monitor the accuracy of reporting on sensitive issues such as drug use and crime. Despite these safeguards, it is not possible to claim that there was no misrepresentation by any of the patients. Yet the critical issue with regard to the interpretation of the results is whether there could have been *differential rates* of misrepresentation between the two groups; which would invalidate the comparisons offered. Since we have no reason to believe that one group of patients was more or less likely to misrepresent, we feel the data collected are reliable and that the results are worthy of consideration.

A final issue in determining the value of these data is the choice of the follow-up interval. There has been discussion about the appropriate or optimal point at which to evaluate treatment effects, with prior workers using intervals ranging from one to 24 months. Our choice of seven months following treatment admission (typically six months following program discharge) was in part based upon our earlier work over the past fifteen years suggesting that approximately 60% to 80% of those patients who relapse following treatment, do so within three to four months after discharge.[16] Finally, since many of the patients who do relapse return to treatment, later follow-up evaluations of a single treatment episode may become contaminated by the effects of subsequent treatments. To our knowledge there is no optimum point at which to evaluate treatment effects and multiple evaluations are therefore preferable. Thus, we suggest that while earlier or later follow-up assessments are important and appropriate, the six-month evaluations provided here also offer one appropriate indication of treatment effects.

CONCLUSION

In conclusion, we believe that the findings presented here offer an initial but important indication of what makes "intensive" outpatient treatment intensive– and what effects this level of intensity has on substance abuse patients as compared with the nature, duration and intensity of services offered in "traditional" outpatient programs. In this regard, it must be admitted that we were disappointed to find that these freestanding "intensive" programs were more intensive *only* in terms of the number of alcohol and drug focused counseling services offered to patients; but not with regard to any other medical or psychosocial services. This may seem to be precisely what should be expected in light of the fact that the patients were admitted for primary problems of alcohol and/or cocaine dependence. In this regard it may be argued that the "related" problems observed in these patients were simply the result of alcohol and drug use– and that with sufficient intensity of services directed at this "root problem" the other "related" problems will also ameliorate. In fact, there is some evidence for this argument in the outcome data shown in Table 4. However, it must be remembered that it was typically the severity of the "related" medical, and social problems of the IO patients that made them unsuitable for traditional outpatient care. Given this situation, we expected to see some significant level of therapeutic focus upon these medical, psychiatric and social problems as part of the rehabilitation plan. While the IO programs did provide services to a somewhat larger proportion of patients than the TO programs in a few of these areas, the level of therapeutic intervention was quite low in all areas and significant problems remained in many of these patients at the follow-up, despite substantial reductions in their alcohol and drug use.

In short, we agree that intensive alcohol and drug focused counseling and support services are the minimum conditions *necessary* for effecting broader changes in the personal health and social function problems of these patients. However, we are not persuaded that this type of "intensive" care by itself, is *sufficient* to produce these broader rehabilitative gains. It may be argued that improvements in these personal health and social function areas are beyond the focus of substance abuse treatment programs that are funded with primary healthcare dollars. We disagree with this argument. We consider improvements in the areas of personal health and social function to be both pertinent to the primary treatment mission of substance abuse programs and pertinent to the interests of those who pay for that treatment. First, as has been argued elsewhere[15] these "addiction related" problems are typically the major reason for referral to treatment. We feel that the public has come to expect improvement in the range of important alcohol and drug "related" problems that are major concerns and significant costs to society. Perhaps more importantly from the perspective of the patient, improvement in the personal health and social function domains are often critical to the maintenance of gains in the substance abuse problem area following treatment. Put simply, even those patients who show abstinence from substance use following treatment–but continue to have unresolved employment, medical, family and/or psychiatric problems–are at significant risk for early relapse.[19-27]

Thus for both the long range goals of society and the individual goals of the patients, we believe that there is a need for treatment strategies that can be effective in addressing the personal health and social function of substance abuse patients as well as their pressing public health and public safety threats. In this regard we are persuaded by the growing body of research showing that professional services focused upon these related areas–*in conjunction with* ongoing alcohol and drug counseling–offer the best chance of more pervasive and more long-lasting rehabilitation.[19-27] As pressures to contain costs of health care increase and as managed care organizations respond to these pressures by reducing the intensity and duration of treatment episodes and the availability of supportive or "wrap around services" such as employment counseling, psychological counseling and family therapy, it is likely that "intensive" outpatient care will be even less intensive. Since the pressures to reduce health care costs will likely continue and since the present report represents only an initial and certainly imperfect examination of this issue, we will return to the issues of the comparative cost-effectiveness of intensive outpatient treatment and other forms of substance abuse treatment in future studies.

REFERENCES

1. Health Policy Report, Medicaid and Managed Care. *The New England Journal of Medicine*, 1995.

2. Mechanic D., Schlesinger M., and McAlpine D.D. Management of mental health and substance abuse services: State of the art and early results. *The Milbank Quarterly,* 1995, 73(1), 19-56.

3. Institute of Medicine *Broadening the Base of Treatment for Alcohol Problems* Washington, D.C., National Academy of Sciences Press, 1990.

4. Hayashida M., Alterman A.I., McLellan A.T., O'Brien C.P., Purtill J., and Volpicelli J. Comparative effectiveness and costs of inpatient and outpatient medical alcohol detoxification, *New Eng. J. Med.* 1989, 320: 358-365.

5. McCrady B.S., Noel N.E., Abrams D.B., Stout R.L., Nelson H.F., and Hay W.M. Comparative effectiveness of three types of spouse involvement in outpatient behavioral alcoholism treatment. *J. Studies on Alcohol,* 1986, 47:459-467.

6. McKay J.R., Alterman A.I., McLellan A.T. and Snider E. Treatment Goals, Continuity of Care and Outcomes in a Day Hospital Substance Abuse Rehabilitation Program. *Am. J. Psychiatry,* 1994, 151(2) 254-259.

7. Alterman A.I., McLellan A.T., O'Brien C.P., August D.S., Snider E.C., Cornish J.C., Droba M., Hall C.P., Raphaelson A. and Schrade F. Effectiveness and Costs of Inpatient Versus Day Hospital Cocaine Rehabilitation. *J. Nerv. Ment. Dis.* 1994, 182: 157-163.

8. Gottheil E., McLellan A.T., and Druley K.A. Laboratory research methodology in the evaluation of alcoholism treatment. In: E. Gottheil et al. (eds.) *Matching Patient Needs and Treatment Methods in Alcohol and Drug Abuse,* Chicago: Charles Thomas Pub., 1981.

9. McLellan A.T., and Durell J. Outcome Evaluation in the Treatment of Substance Use Disorders. In W. Bickel (ed.) *Drug Policy and Human Nature.* Williams and Wilkins, Philadelphia, 1995.

10. American Society of Addiction Medicine. ASAM Patient placement criteria for the treatment of psychoactive substance use disorders. New York, ASAM Press. 1991.

11. McLellan A.T., Luborsky L., O'Brien C.P., and Woody G.E.: An improved diagnostic instrument for substance abuse patients: The Addiction Severity Index. *J. Nerv. & Ment. Diseases,* 1980, 168:26-33.

12. McLellan A.T., Luborsky L., Cacciola J., and Griffith J. New data from the Addiction Severity Index: Reliability and validity in three centers. *J. Nerv. and Ment. Dis.,* 1985, 173: 212-231.

13. McLellan A.T., Cacciola J., Kushner H., Peters R., Smith I., and Pettinati H. The Fifth Edition of the Addiction Severity Index: Cautions, additions and normative data. *J. Substance Abuse Treatment,* 1992, 9(5): 461-480.

14. McLellan A.T., Alterman A.I., Woody G.E., and Metzger D. A quantitative measure of substance abuse treatments: The Treatment Services Review. *J. Nervous & Mental Disease,* 1992, 180:100-109.

15. McLellan A.T. and Weisner C. Achieving the public health potential of substance abuse treatment: Implications for Patient Referral, Treatment "Matching" and Outcome Evaluation. In W. Bickel and R. DeGrandpre (eds.) *Drug Policy and Human Nature.* Wilkins and Wilkins, Philadelphia, 1996, pp. 187-230.

16. McLellan A.T., Woody G.E., Alterman A.I., Metzger D.S., McKay J., Alterman A.I. and O'Brien C.P. Evaluating the Effectiveness of Addiction Treatments: Reasonable Expectations, Appropriate Comparisons *Milbank Quarterly,* 1995, in Press.

17. Hubbard R.L., Marsden M.E., Rachal J.V., Harwood H.J., Cavanaugh E.R. and Ginzburg H.M. *Drug Abuse Treatment: A National Study of Effectiveness.* Chapel Hill: Univ. of North Carolina Press, 1989.

18. Office of Technology Assessment. *The Effectiveness and Costs of Alcoholism Treatment.* Health technology case study 22. Washington D.C., 1983.

19. Ball J.C. and Ross A. *The effectiveness of methadone maintenance treatment: Patients, Programs, Services and Outcomes.* New York, Springer Verlag, 1991.

20. McLellan A.T., Alterman A.I., Metzger D.S., Grissom G., Woody G.E., Luborsky L. and O'Brien C.P. Similarity of Outcome Predictors Across Opiate, Cocaine and Alcohol Treatments: Role of Treatment Services. *J. Clin. Consult. Psychol.,* 1994, 62 (6): 1141-1158.

21. Higgins S.T., Delaney D.D., Budney A.J., Bickel W.K., Hughes J.R., Foerg F., Fenwick J.W. A behavioral approach to achieving initial cocaine abstinence. *Am. J. Psychiat.,* 1991, 148:1218-1224.

22. McCrady B.S., Noel N.E., Abrams D.B., Stout R.L., Nelson H.F., and Hay W.M. Comparative effectiveness of three types of spouse involvement in outpatient behavioral alcoholism treatment. *J. Studies on Alcohol,* 1986, 47:459-467.

23. Stanton M.D. and Todd T. *The Family Therapy of Drug Abuse and Addiction.* New York, Guilford Press, 1982.

24. McLellan A.T., Arndt I.O., Woody G.E., Metzger D. Psychosocial Services in Substance Abuse Treatment?: A dose-ranging study of psychosocial services. *J. Am. Med. Assn.,* 1993, 269(15):1953-1959.

25. Carroll, K.M., Rounsaville, B.J., Gordon, L.T., Nich, C., Jatlow, P., Bisighini, R.M. and Gawin, F.H. Psychotherapy and pharmacotherapy for ambulatory cocaine abusers. *Arch. Gen. Psychiat.* 1994, 51:177-187.

26. Woody G.E., Luborsky L., McLellan A.T. and O'Brien C.P. Psychotherapy for opiate addicts: Does it help? *Arch Gen Psychiatry,* 1983, 40:639-645.

27. French M.T., Dennis M.L., McDougal G.L., Karountzos G.T. and Hubbard R.L. Training and employment programs in methadone treatment: Client needs and desires. *Journal of Substance Abuse Treatment,* 1992, 9:293-303.

SELECTIVE GUIDE TO CURRENT REFERENCE SOURCES ON TOPICS DISCUSSED IN THIS ISSUE

Intensive Outpatient Treatment for the Addictions

Lynn Kasner Morgan, MLS

Each issue of *Journal of Addictive Diseases* features a section offering suggestions on where to look for further information on included topics. The intent is to guide readers to selective substantive sources of current information.

Some published reference works utilize designated terminology (controlled vocabularies) which must be used to find material on topics of interest. For these, a sample of available search terms has been indicated to assist the reader in accessing appropriate sources

Lynn Kasner Morgan is Assistant Professor of Medical Education, Assistant Dean for Information Resources and Systems, and Director of the Gustave L. and Janet W. Levy Library of the Mount Sinai Medical Center, Inc., One Gustave L. Levy Place, New York, NY 10029-6574.

[Haworth co-indexing entry note]: "Selective Guide to Current Reference Sources on Topics Discussed in This Issue." Morgan, Lynn Kasner. Co-published simultaneously in *Journal of Addictive Diseases* (The Haworth Medical Press, an imprint of The Haworth Press, Inc.) Vol. 16, No. 2, 1997, pp. 85-96; and: *Intensive Outpatient Treatment for the Addictions* (ed: Edward Gottheil, and Barry Stimmel) The Haworth Medical Press, an imprint of The Haworth Press, Inc., 1997, pp. 85-96. Single or multiple copies of this article are available for a fee from The Haworth Document Delivery Service [1-800-342-9678, 9:00 a.m. - 5:00 p.m. (EST). E-mail address: getinfo@ haworth.com].

for his/her purposes. Other reference tools use keywords or free text terms from the title of the document, the abstract, and the name of any responsible agency or conference. In searching using keywords, be sure to look under all possible synonyms to retrieve the concept in question.

An asterisk (*) appearing before a published source indicates that all or part of that source is in machine-readable form and can be accessed through an online database search. Database searching is recommended for retrieving sources of information that coordinate multiple variables, concepts, or subject areas. Most health sciences libraries offer database services which can include mediated online searching, access to locally mounted datafiles, front-end software packages, and CD-ROM technology. Searching can also be done from one's office or home with subscriptions to database service vendors and microcomputers equipped with modems.

Interactive electronic communications systems, such as electronic mail, discussion groups, bulletin boards, and receiving and transferring files are available through the Internet, which offers timely and global information resources in all disciplines, including the health sciences. Some groups which might be of interest are: ALCOHOL (ALCOHOL@LMUACAD), DRUG ABUSE (DRUGABUS@UMAB), 12STEP@TRWRB.DSD.COM and ADDICTION MEDICINE (MAJORDOMO@AVOCADO.PC.HELSINKI.FI). The National Clearinghouse for Alcohol and Drug Information Center for Substance Abuse Prevention maintains PREVline, a bulletin board for alcohol and drug information. Information from PREVLINE is available throught the Internet at www.health.org and a recent search included such things as results of the 1995 National Household Survey on Drug Abuse. There are also many sites with World Wide Web pages which can be reached by individuals with a Web browser such as Mosaic or Netscape. Netscape "net search" allows searching with many different web search engines. Suggested starting points are http://www.yahoo.com/health, Web Crawler searching tool http://webcrawler.com or World Wide Web Worm http://wwwmcb.cs.colorado.edu/home/mcbryan/www.html. Other sites to try include: Web of Addictions at http://www.well.com/user/woa; American Psychological Association Division of Pharmacology and Substance Abuse at http://charlotte.med.nyu.edu/woodr/div28.html;

and Online AA resources at http://www.recovery.org. The amount of information available on the Internet increases daily and attention should be given to the author/provider of the information, which ranges from highly respected institutions to individuals with a home computer and a desire to "publish."

Readers are encouraged to consult their librarians for further assistance before undertaking research on a topic.

Suggestions regarding the content and organization of this section are welcome and should be sent to the author.

1. INDEXING AND ABSTRACTING SOURCES

Place of publication, publisher, start date, frequency of publication, and brief descriptions are noted.

*Biological Abstracts (1926-) and *Biological Abstracts/RRM* (v.18, 1980-). Philadelphia, BioSciences Information Service, semimonthly. Reports on worldwide research in the life sciences.

> See: Concept headings for abstracts, such as behavioral biology, pharmacology, psychiatry, public health, and toxicology sections.

> See: Keyword-in-context subject index.

*Chemical Abstracts. Columbus, Ohio, American Chemical Society, 1907- , weekly. A key to the world's literature of chemistry and chemical engineering, including serial publications, proceedings and edited collections, technical reports, dissertations, new book and audiovisual materials announcements, and patent documents.

> See: *Index Guide* for cross-referencing and indexing policies.

> See: *General Subject Index* terms, such as drug dependence, drug-drug interactions, drug tolerance.
> See: Keyword subject indexes.

*Dissertation Abstracts International. Section A. The Humanities and Social Sciences and *Section B. The Sciences and Engineering.* Ann Arbor, Mich., University Microfilms, v.30, 1969/70- , monthly. Includes author-prepared abstracts of doctoral dissertations from 500 participating institutions throughout North America and the world. A separate section contains European dissertations.

See: Keyword subject index.

Excerpta Medica. Amsterdam, The Netherlands, Excerpta Medica Foundation, 1947- , 42 subject sections.

A major abstracting service covering more than 4,300 biomedical journals. The abstracts, including English summaries for non-English-language articles, appear in one or more of the published subject sections, excluding Section 38, *Adverse Reactions Titles,* which is an index only. Each of the sections has a comprehensive subject index. Since 1978 all the *Excerpta Medica* sections have been available for computer searching in the integrated online file, EMBASE.

Particularly relevant to the topics in this issue are Section 40, *Drug Dependence, Alcohol Abuse and Alcoholism;* and the sections that have addiction, alcoholism, or drug subdivisions: Section 30, *Clinical and Experimental Pharmacology;* Section 32, *Psychiatry;* and Section 17, *Public Health, Social Medicine and Epidemiology.*

Hospital and Health Administration Index. Chicago, American Hospital Association, v. 51, 1995- , three issues per year, with annual cumulations. Published as the primary guide to literature on the organization and administration of hospitals and other health care providers, the financing and delivery of healthcare, the development and implementation of health policy and reform, and health planning and research.

See: *MeSH* terms, such as alcohol drinking; alcoholism, ambulatory care; cocaine; metabolic detoxification; methadone; patient dropouts; substance abuse; substance abuse detection; substance abuse treatment centers; substance dependence; rehabilitation; treatment outcome.

Index Medicus (includes *Bibliography of Medical Reviews*). Bethesda, Md., National Library of Medicine, 1960- , monthly, with annual cumulations. Published as author and subject indexes to more than 3,000 journals in the biomedical sciences. Subject headings are based on the controlled vocabulary or thesaurus, *Medical Subject Headings (MeSH).* Since 1966 it has been produced from the MEDLARS database, which provides more comprehensive retrieval, including keyword access and English-language abstracts, than its printed counterparts: *Index Medicus, International Nursing Index,* and *Index to Dental Literature.*

See: *MeSH* terms, such as alcohol drinking; alcoholism; ambulatory care; cocaine; metabolic detoxification; drug; methadone; narcotic addiction; patient dropouts; substance abuse; substance abuse treatment centers; substance dependence; treatment outcome.

Index to Scientific Reviews. Philadelphia, Institute for Scientific Information, 1974- , semiannual.

See: Permuterm keyword subject index.

See: Citation index.

*International Pharmaceutical Abstracts. Washington, D.C., American Society of Hospital Pharmacists, 1964- , semimonthly. A key to the world's literature of pharmacy.

See: IPA subject terms, such as alcoholism; ambulatory care; controlled substances; cocaine; dependence; drug abuse; drug withdrawal; methadone; opiates.

See: Subject sections: legislation, laws and regulations; sociology, economics and ethics; toxicology.

*Psychological Abstracts. Washington, D.C., American Psychological Association, 1927- , monthly. A compilation of nonevaluative summaries of the world's literature in psychology and related disciplines.

See: Index terms, such as addiction, alcohol abuse; alcoholism; alcohol rehabilitation; cocaine; drug abuse; drug addiction; drug dependency; drug rehabilitation; drug usage; drug usage screening; drug withdrawal; halfway houses; methadone; opiates; outpatient treatment; outpatients; residential care institutions; social issues; treatment outcomes.

*Public Affairs Information Service Bulletin. New York, Public Affairs Information Service, v.55, 1969- , semimonthly. An index to library material in the field of public affairs and public policy published throughout the world.

See: PAIS subject headings, such as alcoholism; cocaine; drug abuse; drug addicts; drugs.

*Science Citation Index. Philadelphia, Institute for Scientific Information, 1961- , bimonthly.

See: Permuterm keyword subject index.

See: Citation index.

Social Planning/Policy & Development Abstracts. San Diego, Calif., Sociological Abstracts, Inc., v.6, 1984- , semiannual.

See: Thesaurus and descriptors listed under *Sociological Abstracts.*

Social Work Abstracts. New York, National Association of Social Workers, v.13, 1977- , quarterly.

See: Subject index.

Sociological Abstracts. San Diego, Calif., Sociological Abstracts, Inc., 1952- , 6 times per year. A collection of nonevaluative abstracts which reflect the world's serial literature in sociology and related disciplines.

See: *Thesaurus of Sociological Indexing Terms.*

See: Descriptors such as addict/addicts/addicted/addictive/addiction; alcohol abuse; alcoholism; cocaine; drinking behavior; drug abuse; drug addiction; drug use; outpatients; residential treatment facilities; substance abuse.

2. CURRENT AWARENESS PUBLICATIONS

Current Contents: Clinical Medicine. Philadelphia, Institute for Scientific Information, v.15, 1987- , weekly.

See: Keyword index.

Current Contents: Life Sciences. Philadelphia, Institute for Scientific Information, v. 10, 1967-, weekly.

See: Keyword index.

Current Contents: Social & Behavioral Sciences. Philadelphia, Institute for Scientific Information, v.6, 1974- , weekly.

See: Keyword index.

3. BOOKS

Medical and Health Care Books and Serials in Print: An Index to Literature in the Health Sciences. New York, R. R. Bowker Co., annual.

See: Library of Congress subject headings, such as alcoholism; cocaine; drug abuse; drugs; hospitals-outpatient services.

National Library of Medicine Current Catalog. Bethesda, Md., National Library of Medicine, 1966- , quarterly, with annual cumulations.

See: MeSH terms as noted in Section 1 under *Index Medicus.*

Bellenir, Karen. *Substance Abuse Sourcebook.* Detroit, Omnigraphics, 1996.

O'Brien, Robert [and others]. The Encyclopedia of Drug Abuse. 2nd ed. New York, Facts on File, c1992.

Stimmel, Barry [and others]. *The Facts About Drug Use: Coping with Drug Use in Your Family, at Work, in Your Community.* Mount Vernon, N.Y., Consumers' Union, c1991.

Substance Abuse: The Nation's Number One Health Problem. Key Indicators for Policy. Princeton, N.J., Robert Wood Johnson Foundation, 1993.

Kinney, Jean. *Clinical Manual of Substance Abuse.* St. Louis, Mosby, 1996.

World Health Organization Catalogue: New Books. Geneva, World Health Organization, semiannual (supplements *World Health Organization Publications* and includes periodicals).

See Also: http://www.who.org

4. U.S. GOVERNMENT PUBLICATIONS

Alcohol and Other Drug Thesaurus: A Guide to Concepts and Terminology in Substance Abuse and Addiction (AOD Thesaurus). Rockville, Md., National Institute on Alcohol Abuse and Alcoholism, 1993.

See: Title keyword index.

Monthly Catalog of United States Government Publications. Washington, D.C., U.S. Government Printing Office, 1895- , monthly.

See: Keyword index.

See Also: http://www.access.gpo.gov

5. ONLINE BIBLIOGRAPHIC DATABASES

Only those databases which have no print counterparts are included in this section. Print sources which have online database equivalents are noted throughout this guide by the asterisk (*) which appears before the title. If you do not have direct access to these databases, consult your librarian for assistance.

ALCOHOL AND ALCOHOL PROBLEMS SCIENCE DATABASE: ETOH (National Institute on Alcohol Abuse and Alcoholism, Rockville, Md.).

>   Use: Keywords.

ALCOHOL INFORMATION FOR CLINICIANS AND EDUCATORS (Project Cork Institute, Dartmouth Medical School, Hanover, N.H.).

>   Use: Keywords.

>   See Also: http://www.dartmouth.edu/dms/cork

AMERICAN STATISTICS INDEX (ASI) (Congressional Information Services, Inc., Washington, D.C.).

>   Use: Keywords.

DRUG INFORMATION FULLTEXT (American Society of Hospital Pharmacists, Bethesda, Md.).

>   Use: Keywords.

DRUGINFO AND ALCOHOL USE AND ABUSE (Hazelden Foundation, Center City, Minn., and Drug Information Service Center, College of Pharmacy, University of Minnesota, Minneapolis, Minn.).

>   Use: Keywords.

>   See Also: http://www.hazelden.org

LEXIS (LESIX-NESIS, Dayton, Ohio).

>   Use: Guide library.

MAGAZINE INDEX (Information Access Co., Foster City, Calif.).

> Use: Keywords.

MENTAL HEALTH ABSTRACTS (MHA) (IFI/Plenum Data Co., Wilmington, NC).

> Use: Keywords.

NATIONAL NEWSPAPER INDEX (Information Access Co., Foster City, Calif.).

> Use: Keywords.

NTIS (Bibliographic Data Base, U.S. National Technical Information Service, Springfield, Va.).

> Use: Keywords.

PSYCINFO (American Psychological Association, Washington, D.C.).

> Use: Keywords.

WESTLAW (West Publishing Co., St. Paul, Minn.).

> Use: Keywords.

6. HANDBOOKS, DIRECTORIES, GRANT SOURCES, ETC.

Annual Register of Grant Support. Wilmette, Ill., National Register Pub. Co., annual.

> See: Internal medicine; medicine; pharmacology, psychiatry, psychology, mental health sections.

> See: Subject index.

*Biomedical Index to PHS-Supported Research. Bethesda, Md., National Institutes of Health, Division of Research Grants, annual.

> See: Subject index.

Database Directory. White Plains, N.Y., Knowledge Industry Publications in cooperation with the American Society for Information Science, annual.

> See: Subject index.

Directory of Research Grants. Phoenix, Ariz., Oryx Press, annual.

> See: Subject index terms, such as alcohol/alcoholism, education, drugs/drug abuse, health promotion.

Encyclopedia of Associations. Detroit, Gale Research Co., annual (occasional supplements between editions).

> See: Subject index.

Foundation Directory. New York, The Foundation Center, biennial (updated between editions by *Foundation Directory Supplement*).

> See: Index of foundations.

> See: Index of foundations by state and city.

> See: Index of donors, trustees, and administrators.

> See: Index of fields of interest.

> See Also: http://www.fancenter.org

Health Hotlines: Toll-Free Numbers from DIRLINE. Bethesda, Md., National Library of Medicine, biennial.

Information Industry Directory. Detroit, Gale Research Co., annual.

Nolan, Kathleen Lopez. *Gale Directory of Databases.* Detroit, Gale Research, Inc., 1995.

Roper, Fred W. and Jo Anne Boorkman. *Introduction to Reference Sources in the Health Sciences.* 3rd ed. Chicago, Medical Library Association, c1994.

The SALIS Directory: Substance Abuse Librarians and Information Specialists. 2nd ed. Berkeley, Calif., Alcohol Research Group, Medical Research Institute of San Francisco and University of California, Berkeley, 1991.

Statistics Sources. 19th ed. Detroit, Gale Research Inc., 1996.

7. *JOURNAL LISTINGS*

**The Serials Directory. An International Reference Book.* Birmingham, Ebsco Publishing, annual (supplemented by quarterly updates).

**Ulrich's International Periodicals Directory, Now Including Irregular Serials & Annuals.* New York, R. R. Bowker Co., annual (updated between editions by *Ulrich's Quarterly).*

> See: Subject categories, such as drug abuse and alcoholism, medical sciences, pharmacy and pharmacology, psychology, public health and safety.

8. *AUDIOVISUAL PROGRAMS*

The Directory of Medical Video Programs. Hawthorne, N.J., Ridge Publishing Co., 1990.

**National Library of Medicine Audiovisuals Catalog.* Bethesda, Md., National Library of Medicine, 1977-1993, quarterly, with annual cumulations.

> See: *MeSH* terms as noted in Section 1 under *Index Medicus.*

Patient Education Sourcebook. 2v. Saint Louis, Mo., Health Sciences Communications Association, c1985-90.

> See: *MeSH* terms as noted in Section 1 under *Index Medicus.*

9. *GUIDES TO UPCOMING MEETINGS*

Scientific Meetings. San Diego, Calif., Scientific Meetings Publications, quarterly.

> See: Subject indexes.

> See: Association listing.

World Meetings: Medicine. New York, Macmillan Pub. Co., quarterly.

> See: Keyword index.

See: Sponsor directory and index.

World Meetings: Outside United States and Canada. New York, Macmillan Pub. Co., quarterly.

See: Keyword index.

See: Sponsor directory and index.

World Meetings: United States and Canada. New York, Macmillan Pub. Co., quarterly.

See: Keyword index.

See: Sponsor directory and index.

10. PROCEEDINGS OF MEETINGS

Directory of Published Proceedings. Series SEMT. Science/Engineering/Medicine/Technology. Harrison, N.Y., InterDok Corp., v.3, 1967- , monthly, except July-August, with annual cumulations.

Index to Scientific and Technical Proceedings. Philadelphia, Institute for Scientific Information, 1978- , monthly with semiannual cumulations.

11. SPECIALIZED RESEARCH CENTERS

Medical Research Centres. Harlow, Essex, Longman, biennial.

International Research Centers Directory. Detroit, Gale Research Co., annual.

Research Centers Directory. Detroit, Gale Research Co., annual (updated by *New Research Centers*).

12. SPECIAL LIBRARY COLLECTIONS

Directory of Special Libraries and Information Centers. Detroit, Gale Research Co., annual (updated by *New Special Libraries*).

Index

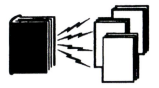

Haworth
DOCUMENT DELIVERY
SERVICE

This valuable service provides a single-article order form for any article from a Haworth journal.

- *Time Saving:* No running around from library to library to find a specific article.
- *Cost Effective:* All costs are kept down to a minimum.
- *Fast Delivery:* Choose from several options, including same-day FAX.
- *No Copyright Hassles:* You will be supplied by the original publisher.
- *Easy Payment:* Choose from several easy payment methods.

Open Accounts Welcome for . . .
- Library Interlibrary Loan Departments
- Library Network/Consortia Wishing to Provide Single-Article Services
- Indexing/Abstracting Services with Single Article Provision Services
- Document Provision Brokers and Freelance Information Service Providers

---

MAIL or *FAX* THIS ENTIRE ORDER FORM TO:

Haworth Document Delivery Service
The Haworth Press, Inc.
10 Alice Street
Binghamton, NY 13904-1580

or FAX: 1-800-895-0582
or CALL: 1-800-342-9678
9am-5pm EST

PLEASE SEND ME PHOTOCOPIES OF THE FOLLOWING SINGLE ARTICLES:
1) Journal Title: _____
   Vol/Issue/Year:_____ Starting & Ending Pages:_____
Article Title:_____
_____

2) Journal Title: _____
   Vol/Issue/Year: _____ Starting & Ending Pages:_____
Article Title:_____
_____

3) Journal Title: _____
   Vol/Issue/Year: _____ Starting & Ending Pages:_____
Article Title:_____
_____

4) Journal Title: _____
   Vol/Issue/Year: _____ Starting & Ending Pages:_____
Article Title:_____
_____

(See other side for Costs and Payment Information)

COSTS: Please figure your cost to order quality copies of an article.

1. Set-up charge per article: $8.00
         ($8.00 × number of separate articles) _____

2. Photocopying charge for each article:
         1-10 pages: $1.00 _____

         11-19 pages: $3.00 _____

         20-29 pages: $5.00 _____

         30+ pages: $2.00/10 pages _____

3. Flexicover (optional): $2.00/article _____

4. Postage & Handling: US: $1.00 for the first article/
         $.50 each additional article _____

         Federal Express: $25.00 _____

         Outside US: $2.00 for first article/
         $.50 each additional article _____

5. Same-day FAX service: $.35 per page _____

               GRAND TOTAL: _____

METHOD OF PAYMENT: (please check one)

❑ Check enclosed   ❑ Please ship and bill. PO # _____
      (sorry we can ship and bill to bookstores only! All others must pre-pay)

❑ Charge to my credit card: ❑ Visa; ❑ MasterCard; ❑ Discover;
      ❑ American Express;

Account Number: _____ Expiration date: _____

Signature: ✗ _____

Name: _____ Institution: _____

Address: _____

_____

City: _____ State: _____ Zip: _____

Phone Number: _____ FAX Number: _____

MAIL or *FAX* THIS ENTIRE ORDER FORM TO:

Haworth Document Delivery Service	**or FAX:** 1-800-895-0582
The Haworth Press, Inc.	**or CALL:** 1-800-342-9678
10 Alice Street	9am-5pm EST)
Binghamton, NY 13904-1580	

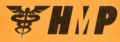